D1178306

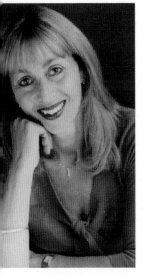

Maryon Stewart studied preventive dentistry and nutrition at St George's Hospital in London and worked as a counsellor with nutritional doctors in England for four years. At the beginning of 1984, she set up the PMT Advisory Service, which has subsequently helped thousands of women worldwide. In 1987, she launched the Women's Nutritional Advisory Service, and in 2003, the Natural Health Advisory Service, which now provides broader help to people of all ages around the world. As a result of her work, she was voted in the top 100 most influential women in the UK in a Good Housekeeping survey.

Maryon is the author of the best-selling books, The Real Life Plan, The Phyto Factor, Cruising Through the Menopause, No More PMS, Beat Sugar Craving, The Zest for Life Plan and Healthy Parents, Healthy Baby. She is the co-author of No More IBS, Beat PMS Cookbook, Every Woman's Health Guide and The Natural Health Bible. She is also the author of The Model Plan, published while working as the nutritional consultant to the British Channel 4 program, Model Behavior.

Maryon has co-written several medical papers and written for many national magazines and newspapers, including House & Garden, Healthy Eating, The Sunday Express Magazine, The Daily Mirror, The Daily Mail and The Express. She has been an adviser and contributor to Good Health Magazine and on the expert panel for Top Santé magazine and First Steps. She is currently a consultant and regular contributor to Health and Fitness magazine and contributes regularly to many other magazines and newspapers.

Maryon has worked extensively on radio, including her own weekly health and nutrition program, and has contributed to over 1,000 radio programs. She has appeared on dozens of TV programs and contributed to many TV series. She frequently lectures to both the public and the medical profession. Maryon has four children and lives in Brighton, England.

Beat Menopause Naturally by Maryon Stewart
www.askmaryonstewart.com
www.naturalmenopause.com

Copyright © 2006 text Maryon Stewart

Edited by Kris Abbey & Jane Garton

Designed by Kris Abbey of Commotion Pty Ltd

Photography by Katrina Sutherland of beanshoot
Several food images supplied by Teresa Cutter (Bite Me, Body+Soul)

Although every effort has been made to ensure the contents of this book are accurate, it must not be treated as a substitute for qualified
medical advice. Always consult a qualified medical practitioner. Neither the author nor the publisher can be held responsible for any loss or
claim arising out of the use or misuse of the suggestions made or for a failure to take medical advice. Always consult your practitioner before
adopting any of the advice contained in this publication. All liability arising directly or indirectly from the use of, or for any omissions in, the
information given is expressly disclaimed

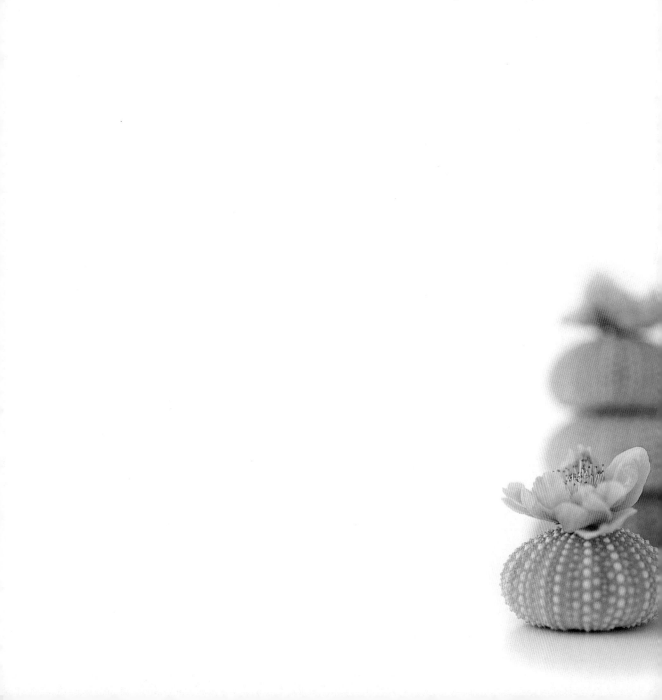

To the wonderful women who were willing to share
their very personal stories in our film,
in this book, and on our web site in the hope that they
will help millions of other women
and their families around the world:

Sarah Adams
Helen Benton
Eleanor Burns
Lynn Carr
Jennifer Colby
Jean Cunningham
Jo De Lisle
Mairin Gallagher
Rosanna Haslam
Ann Higgins
Zoe Howes
Anne Keene
Jean Krane
Donna Lothian
Cherie Lunghi
Sharyn McLaughlin
Diana Moran
Marva Morrison
Denise Pemberton
Merle Shapiro
Gladys Sellars
Joanne Simms
Kate Waters
Barbara York

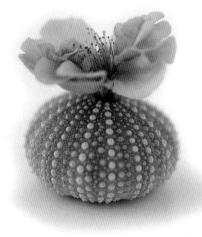

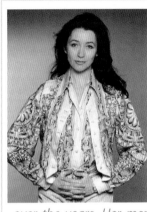

Cherie's Story

Cherie Lunghi is a very well-known and talented actress who has appeared in many US and UK films and TV documentaries over the years. Her menopause symptoms began suddenly and were disrupting her life when she came to see me in the clinic.

I was taken by surprise by my menopause symptoms and I admit it was somewhat of a shock to have reached that stage in my life. I found myself suddenly suffering appalling anxiety, I became easily wound up about very small things and was left feeling desperately tired as a result of my sleep being disrupted by the night sweats. When I had a hot flash when I was working, I couldn't concentrate on what my director was saying, which I found both disconcerting and embarrassing. Maryon was recommended by a friend in whom I confided and thankfully it was only three or four weeks after seeing her that I started feeling better. I cut out caffeine and used decaffeinated drinks and cut back on alcohol as every time I had a glass of wine I began flashing. I began using soy milk and yogurt instead of dairy and that was a huge help too. Plus I took the supplements Gynovite, Promensil and Cardiozen and made sure I took regular exercise. I hurt my back shortly after starting Maryon's program, so I had some acupuncture which I definitely think helped as well. I feel 500% better now. I'm much more energetic, I haven't got any of the symptoms and I feel like a completely different person, which is truly wonderful.

Acknowledgments

Until now, I only ever dreamed of launching a Kit that would be a true reflection of our successful Menopause Program. This program has helped millions of women all around the world overcome their symptoms of menopause and learn how to improve their long-term health prospects. I truly thank the men and women who believed enough in this project to fund and support it.

Although this is my 25th book (and I certainly never dreamed I would get to number 25!), this one is special and different in its own way. First, it is the workbook to complement our DVD, Get Fit for Midlife and Manage Menopause Naturally. Second, it will be available to women all around the world as part of the Natural Menopause Kit, so menopause will come to represent 'a new beginning' rather than 'the beginning of the end'!

When it came to dedicating this book, I felt it clearly had to be dedicated to those women who unselfishly put their personal details in the public arena in a bid to help others. Again, my heartfelt thanks to them.

My thanks also to the researchers around the world who have shared their work and made it possible for us to devise such a workable, enjoyable and effective program to sail through menopause.

I am also very grateful to Jane Garton for her contribution and editing skills, Sue Fisher Hendry for contributing to the section on reframing attitudes, Katherine Burke for helping with medical references, Kris Abbey for editing and wonderful design and Anita Williams, Linda Coffey, Dana Whiteley and Sue Fisher Hendry for proofreading and adapting this book for each territory.

On the home front, I'm enormously grateful to my two children who have not yet flown the nest, Hester and Simeon, for being willing to share me and put up with my utter preoccupation while I pulled this project together. My deepest gratitude goes to my two grown children, Phoebe and Chesney, who freely gave professional advice to help me shape the project in its early stages. Knowing the far-reaching health benefits as we all do, we think it was well worth the effort.

Maryon Stewart, January 2007

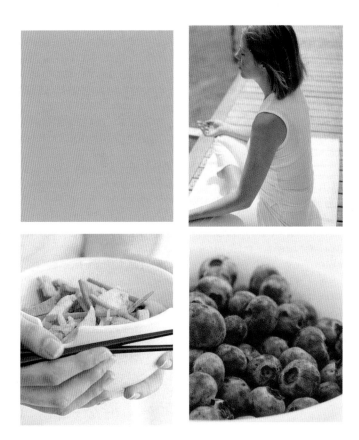

contents

"This is a time of growth, a time for women to embrace who they really are. Ideally a woman should be wanting to spend much less time hanging around looking for the fountain of youth and a lot more time luxuriating and bathing in the waters of wisdom."

Sue Fisher Hendry

Foreword

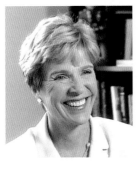

Every woman is emotionally, physically and spiritually different. So are their experiences with menopause. Many women welcome menopause as a relief from monthly periods and the problems related to the menstrual cycle, including the need for contraception. Other women regret the end of their reproductive years or view menopause as a loss of their youth. Some women never experience a hot flash or night sweat, while other women find their quality of life is seriously compromised by hot flashes and night sweats.

Menopause is not a disease. It is a normal occurrence in the life of every woman who lives long enough to experience it. Regardless of the symptoms experienced before, during or after menopause, it is a good time for a woman to take stock of her health and make changes that will help her to live a long, healthy and happy life. After all, we can now expect to live almost as long after menopause as before menopause.

What women choose to do about their symptoms, or their health, at menopause is also unique to every woman. Whether or not a woman needs, or chooses, to use hormone therapy, all women should know what they need to do to feel better—perhaps even better than before menopause.

This Natural Menopause Kit will help women understand what to expect at menopause. More importantly, it provides a host of options for women to choose from to make decisions that will help them stay healthy and vital in the ensuing years. Health and vitality is not something that comes in a bottle. It is reliant on the choices we make regarding our diet, exercise regimen and other behaviours. The Natural Menopause Kit helps guide consumers in making those healthy choices.

Susan Wysocki, President of the National Association of Nurse Practitioners in Women's Health, USA

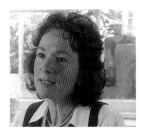

The menopause is a milestone in every woman's life. We may greet it with relief as an end to the tyranny of premenstrual syndrome, contraception, periods and migraines. Or we may regret the loss of fertility and the acknowledgment of aging. Most women feel a mixture of emotions, but what we really want is information about the process. We want to know what options are available so we can make informed decisions about our future health and feel comfortable with our choices. This book is designed to help women do this.

Even at the height of the popularity of Hormone Replacement Therapy (HRT), 70% of women opted not to take prescribed HRT, preferring to go though the process 'naturally'. Since the publication in 2003 of two huge research studies on women's health (the Women's Health Initiative study from the USA and the Million Women Study from the UK), there have been serious concerns about the breast cancer risks associated with estrogen+progestogen HRT. Some women still take HRT and have made that evidence-based choice in conjunction with their doctor. Most women prefer to try to keep healthy and stay fit without medication.

This book explains all the symptoms of menopause and the related health issues you might expect in the future. It summarizes all the information needed to keep yourself fit and healthy, and the useful diet, exercise and lifestyle advice is perfect for anyone wanting to turn over a new leaf.

Dr Sally Hope, FRCGP DRCGP

part one

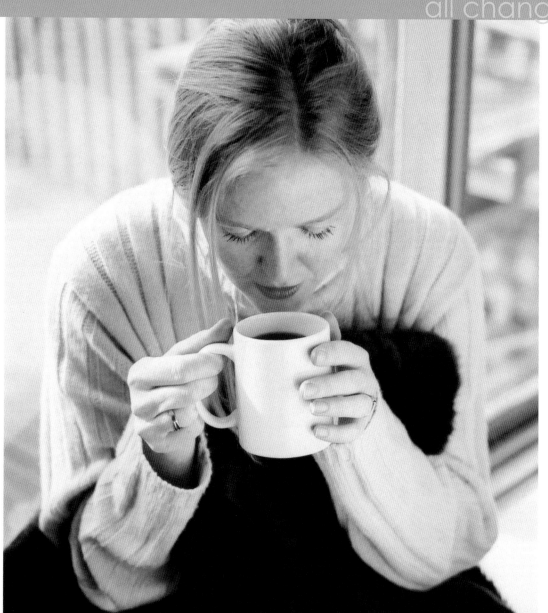

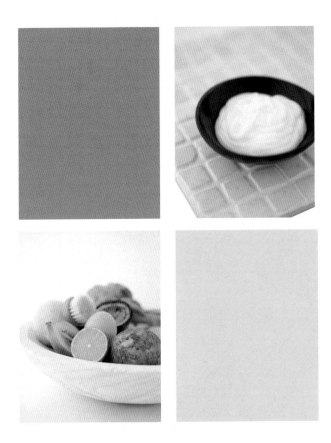

the beginning

You may be nearing the menopause, you may have already reached it, or you may even be coming out the other end and wondering how to protect your heart, bones and memory in the long-term. You probably don't know which way to turn, as there is so much conflicting advice out there. Should you just put up with the symptoms, should you go on Hormone Replacement Therapy (HRT) although you don't particularly want to, or should you try some of the many natural and herbal supplements available, and if so which ones? And what if you're already taking HRT – should you continue or should you come off because of the long-term implications?

You have every reason to be confused. The newspapers and media, not to mention doctors and nurses, are full of advice on the best ways to approach this important stage in your life, yet they don't always agree with each other and many of the options offered are not even vaguely scientifically based.

The most popular treatment for menopausal symptoms over the past 20 years has been HRT. However, several major international HRT studies have now been aborted due to the increased risk for participants of serious medical conditions, such as heart disease, stroke, thrombosis, breast cancer and ovarian cancer. Understandably, many women are now looking for an alternative treatment to HRT.

19

The Natural Menopause Program is a scientifically based, natural, proven alternative to hormone treatment. Over the past 20 years, we at the Natural Health Advisory Service (NHAS) have pioneered this simple, workable and enjoyable program to help alleviate symptoms during the years leading up to your last period and beyond. The program is based on sound research and extensive clinical practice, and the success rate, within a matter of months, astounds most of our patients and is a constant source of satisfaction for our dedicated team of health professionals.

Many years of working with menopausal women at the NHAS (including several important research projects we undertook to measure levels of nutrients in women at different stages of their lives) has led me to realize that falling levels of estrogen are not the only trigger of menopausal symptoms. There are other things to blame.

Factors such as diet and lifestyle play a part. Pregnancy, breast-feeding and physical and mental stress also take their toll on our wellbeing. Levels of some nutrients drop naturally as we age. Taking all this into account, it's not surprising that by the time many women reach menopause, they are firing on two cylinders instead of four. As a result, if they are not in a good nutritional or physiological state, their menopausal symptoms and long-term health prospects are likely to be more severe.

Once we realize that menopausal symptoms are not all related to falling levels of estrogen, and that other physical and mental factors are involved, it follows that any successful program must encompass all three areas. So it's no coincidence that our Natural Menopause Program encompasses all these factors with consistently fantastic results. A recent survey showed that over 91% of women who followed our program felt that their estrogen withdrawal symptoms were under control within five months, while their other physical and mental symptoms had significantly improved.

Tried and Tested

The trick is to find the right program for you, which allows you to control your symptoms, rather than allowing them to control you. This is where the Natural Menopause Kit can really help you. It contains all the tried and tested secrets of our highly successful program. It shows you how to overhaul your diet and other aspects of your life and provides a multi-pronged attack to help overcome your symptoms and, more importantly, keep yourself in great shape in the long-term.

Self-Assessment

I have devised a series of questionnaires that enable you to assess which areas of your life need addressing. It could be that you have low levels of important nutrients, which are affecting your mood and energy levels, or fluctuating levels of hormones, which are making you hot and bothered, or you're not exercising enough, you have too much stress in your life, you have low libido or you're just generally feeling below par.

All you have to do is take the simple tests to identify where your main problems lie and get going on your own individual menopause plan. Based on your results, I will show you how to tailor your plan to suit your own specific needs, tastes and budget.

"I feel 500% better now. I'm more energetic, I haven't got any of the symptoms and I feel like a completely different person, which is truly wonderful."
Cherie Lunghi

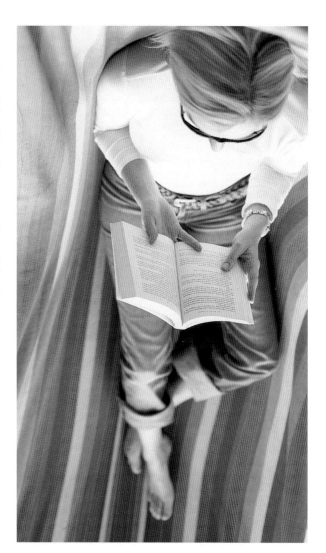

So let's get started...

To determine whether or not you are ready to undergo the program, do this quick test. Check yes or no to the following questions. Make sure you give an honest and spontaneous answer.

	Yes	No
Hot flashes	☐	☐
Night sweats	☐	☐
Vaginal dryness	☐	☐
Anxiety	☐	☐
Irregular or heavy periods	☐	☐
Need the restroom often	☐	☐
Stress incontinence	☐	☐
Forgetfulness	☐	☐
Depression	☐	☐
Loss of confidence	☐	☐
Lack of concentration	☐	☐
Difficulty sleeping	☐	☐
Aches and pains in joints	☐	☐
Palpitations	☐	☐
Panic attacks	☐	☐
Headaches	☐	☐
Loss of sex drive	☐	☐
Painful sex	☐	☐
Mood swings	☐	☐
Fatigue	☐	☐
Weight gain	☐	☐
Bloating	☐	☐

What Your Score Means

If you scored more than three 'yes' answers, then working through the Natural Menopause Program will help you devise your own plan to overcome your particular perimenopause or menopause symptoms, and if necessary even provide you with a tried and tested way to wean yourself off HRT without any side-effects.

You can reinstate your self-esteem, rekindle your libido, resurrect your memory, recharge your batteries and regain your zest for life - all in the space of a few short months - by following a program that has helped literally hundreds of thousands of women all over the world during the past 20 years.

"Within six weeks, I felt like a different person. I wasn't spaced out any more. I had no more panic attacks or depression, and I felt I was once more in control of my body. I realized that I'd lost three years of my life!"
Jo De Lisle

22

How the Program Works

To get on the road to a 'new you', fill in the health questionnaires, which you will find in many of the chapters, then turn to page 322 and enter your score. After four months, you will need to reassess your score. Realistically, you need to follow the program for at least four to six months to gain optimum benefit, after which it can be tailored more to your needs to help you stay in control of your health prospects.

As you go through each chapter, make a note of the action points you need to follow, so by the time you have finished Part One of this book, you will have your own personally tailored Natural Menopause Plan. Combine these recommendations with the delicious recipes in Part Three to ensure you meet your body's new nutritional needs. You will also find notes on the nutritional content of food, as well as a list of nutritional supplements that have been medically proven to soothe symptoms and help boost your overall health and wellbeing.

As soon as you start to become aware of your body's individual needs, those everyday irritations - such as hot flashes, night sweats, depression, headaches, aches and pains, insomnia, mood swings and anxiety - will begin to subside. You will also start to lower your risk of suffering many life-disrupting (and often life-threatening) conditions, including heart disease, osteoporosis, many of the estrogen-dependent cancers, kidney problems, memory loss and dementia.

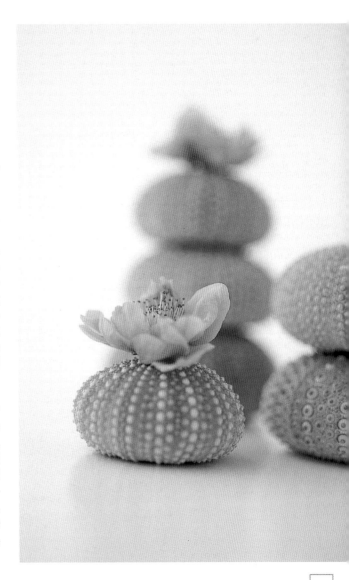

Hillary's Story

Hillary, 49, from London came to the NHAS with severe menopausal symptoms.

<u>*Before*</u>

Hot and cold flashes during the day
Insomnia
Depression
Digestive problems
Sudden weight gain
A feeling of losing her grip on life

<u>*After One Month on the NHAS*</u>
<u>*Menopause Program*</u>

All hot and cold flashes stopped
Less anxiety
Steady weight loss
Better sleep
Better mood

A New You

Having treated hundreds of thousands of women over the years at the Natural Health Advisory Service, I have witnessed so many wonderful transformations as women regain their quality of health, confidence and self-esteem. The women who have so generously shared their experiences for this book are just a few typical examples. Their stories show you that you are not suffering alone and that the end of your symptoms is in sight.

My aim is to inform and educate women by clearly explaining the pros and cons of HRT and to spread the word about the highly successful program pioneered by the NHAS so women everywhere have sufficient information to enable them to make informed choices throughout menopause and beyond. This is your chance to get back in the driver's seat of your life!

Visual Effects

Making the DVD was an enlightening experience on many levels. My patients who took part spent the weekend together while we filmed and they immediately bonded as a group. I never considered the effect that meeting with other women with similar experiences would have on them. When they each contacted me following the weekend, it soon became obvious that it was a life-changing experience they all enjoyed enormously.

Join the Club

When I gave it more thought, I realized there was a need for women around the world to meet and exchange experiences, as well as receive ongoing advice and news, so I decided to start an online community called Maryon Stewart's Lifebay.

If your package includes membership, log on to www.askmaryonstewart.com, click on member's login and enter your password. You will have immediate access to the members' area and can ask me questions and participate in the regular Telephone Workshops. Just check out the workshop dates and send me your questions.

At the same time, you can download The Menopause Newsletter, read helpful articles and tune into our weekly news round-up to hear ground-breaking news and special interviews with experts and guests from all around the world. You will also be able to chat with other women online and compare notes and, through our video diaries, follow the progress of other women going through our program.

If you're not already a member and would like to become one, go to www.askmaryonstewart.com/member and sign up. It is that easy. I wish you a safe passage and I look forward to meeting you all at Lifebay. In the meantime, enjoy the book as it was written with you in mind!

Angela's Story

Angela, 49, from the West Midlands came to the NHAS for an alternative to HRT.

Before

Hot flashes – 'on fire'
Headaches
Fatigue
Constipation
Weight gain (9.5kg)

After 4 Months on the NHAS Menopause Program

Hot flashes gone
No headaches
No constipation
Weight loss (5kg)
Feels like she is back in the driver's seat

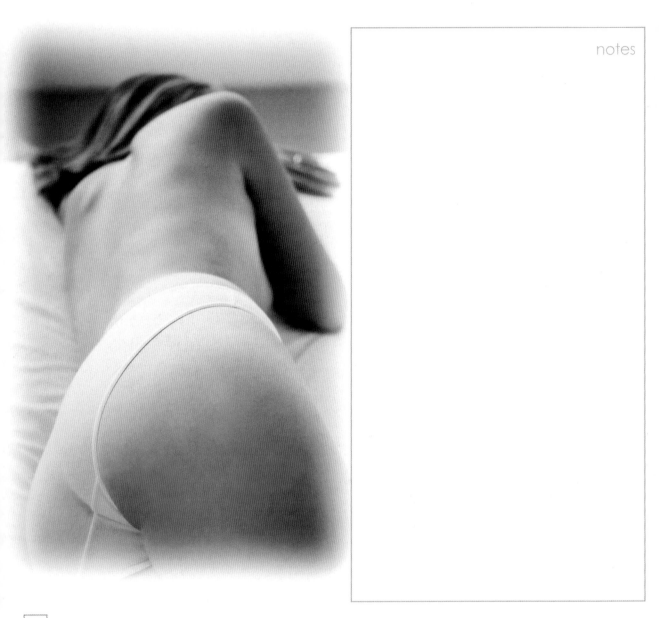

notes

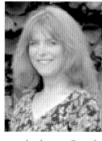

Jo's Story

Jo De Lisle is a retired teacher living with her husband and two sons. She was recovering from a nervous breakdown as a result of extreme harassment in the workplace. By the time she sought help she was suicidal and full of self-disgust and hate.

I first experienced menopausal symptoms four years ago when my periods became more frequent and I started to have hot flashes. I had taken early retirement from work after an unpleasant situation had got out of hand. I felt as though I was going through bereavement, grieving the loss of myself, and had terrible mood swings. My doctor suggested I try HRT.

Almost immediately, I started gaining weight, over 30kg in all - equivalent to four dress sizes! I also started getting headaches, which seemed to last all day and night, and it felt like I had constant PMT. I was bloated and constipated, and I became obsessed with chocolate - some days I ate nothing except blocks of chocolate.

Then one day my friend rang and told me she had seen Maryon Stewart, who had helped her through her severe menopausal symptoms. She lent me one of Maryon's books and begged me to make an appointment to see her. But I was in such a state, I never got around to it. I went through a period of feeling suicidal for three weeks and my husband finally cracked because he couldn't cope. He hit out at our 15-year-old son and it ended with both my sons and my husband crying. I knew I had to seek help before our frustrations became physical.

Maryon listened carefully to my tale of woe and gave me masses of reassurance. I still wasn't convinced, but I knew I had to give her recommendations a try. I came off the HRT and followed the program as best I could.

Within six weeks, I felt like a different person. I wasn't spaced out or foggy any more and I felt I was once more in control of my body. I realized that I'd lost three years of my life!

As the months passed, I felt happier and more positive than I had for years. The weight started to fall off and I began to get back to my normal size. Now I feel calm and happy to the point of feeling bubbly. I look so different that people I know walk by me in the street without recognising me. I feel like I've found a new me. I honestly never thought I would live to see the day when I could lead a normal, happy life again. I am so very grateful to be able to do this again.

"Menopause, rather than being seen as the beginning of the end, should be seen more as a new beginning."

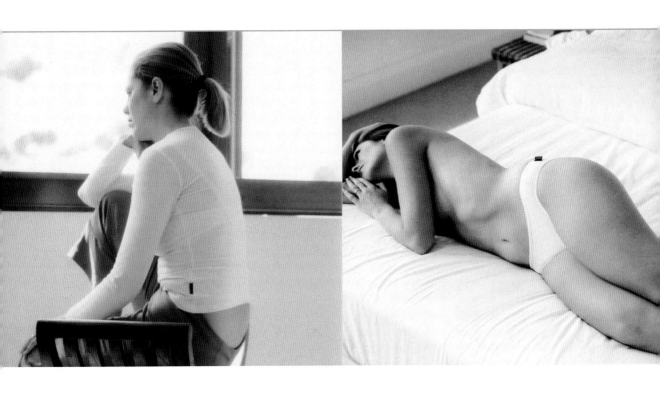

what's happening to me?

One night, out of the blue, you find yourself waking up in a hot sweat. You throw off the covers, even though the room temperature is freezing. At first, this only happens occasionally. But as time goes on, it becomes a nightly occurrence, breaking your sleep and leaving you worn out the next day.

And your days aren't that much better. Increasingly, you start feeling waves of heat rising through your body, often when you get hot or in moments of stress, such as when you're sitting in a traffic jam, in a meeting or on a crowded train. Your periods become erratic and your moods are like those of a teenager. What on earth is going on with you? You're not ill, nor are you going mad. Your body is approaching menopause.

Menopause literally means the last day of your last period, although most of us use the word pretty loosely to describe the various symptoms that we experience in the years before and after this event. It can happen any time between the ages of 45 and 55, with around 51 the average in the US.

In about 1% of women, menopause happens before the age of 40. This is known as premature menopause or premature ovarian failure (POF).

Early Menopause

You are more likely to have a premature menopause if:

- You have your ovaries removed by surgery (oophorectomy), which sometimes happens with a hysterectomy if your ovaries are abnormal or to prevent the spread of endometriosis or ovarian or endometrial cancer

- You have radiotherapy or chemotherapy for treatment of leukemia or cancer

- You have a family history (hereditary genetic cause) or a chromosomal defect

- You smoke. (Research shows smoking is a major factor, with heavy smokers reaching menopause up to two years earlier than non-smokers)

- You had your last child before you were 28

- You have never had children

- You are short or underweight

- Your diet is nutritionally poor

Why Does Menopause Happen?

At birth, our ovaries contain thousands of follicles, or egg sacs, in which egg cells ripen and develop. At puberty, our ovaries start to release an egg each month under the influence of two chemical messengers, or hormones, produced by the pituitary gland in the brain. These two hormones, Follicle Stimulating Hormone (FSH) and Luteinizing Hormone (LH), in turn trigger our ovaries to produce two more hormones, estrogen and progesterone, which are responsible for preparing the lining of our womb for pregnancy. If an egg is not fertilized, estrogen and progesterone levels decline and the egg, together with the build-up of womb lining, is shed in the form of a period.

As you go through your 40s, the supply of eggs you were born with starts to run out and your ovaries stop releasing an egg each month. This means you no longer produce so much progesterone and estrogen. Eventually, your ovaries run out of eggs altogether, progesterone production ceases and estrogen levels fall. Estrogen is required for many bodily functions - not just for reproduction - including strong bones, a sharp mind and a healthy heart, so it is inevitable that you will feel the effects of decreasing estrogen.

The Perimenopause

Your body goes through a series of changes leading up to menopause. These are known collectively as the 'perimenopause' ('peri' meaning 'around'). The first sign that things are on the move is usually a change in the pattern of your periods. They may become irregular, longer or shorter, as well as heavier or in some cases lighter. Other perimenopausal symptoms include hot flashes, night sweats, mood swings, loss of libido, loss of energy, sleepless nights and not being able to concentrate – at first just occasionally, but as time goes by, more and more frequently.

Most of us are unprepared for perimenopause. It may simply bring a degree of unpredictability into your life, since you never know when your period is going to arrive. If you are less fortunate, you may experience a worsening of PMS symptoms, as well as regular mood swings and more 'black' days than you dare to count.

PMS Meets Perimenopause

Premenstrual Syndrome (PMS) is the physical and mental symptoms that can occur just before the arrival of a period, then diminish or disappear shortly afterwards. Most women who suffer from PMS do not enjoy the hormonal roller coaster involved. If your PMS bumps into the start of your menopause symptoms, which is quite common, then you have the worst of both worlds! But fortunately this can be sorted out effectively within a few months.

Studies reveal that PMS is most prevalent in the 30-something age group. So why are we talking about it here in a book on midlife? Well, for some women, PMS never quite goes away. In fact, due to the hormonal instability at this time, PMS can become even worse in perimenopause.

This factor, together with other hormone-related factors, has caused many researchers to attribute PMS to a lack (or excess) of just about any hormone you care to mention! The medical profession does not speak with one voice on this matter. More critical research, however, has found no consistent hormonal abnormality in the majority of PMS sufferers. A more modern understanding is to blame the cause of PMS to the undue sensitivity of the sufferer to the normal hormonal changes that take place in the last half of the cycle. This makes it much easier to see how PMS might fit in with some women's perimenopausal experience.

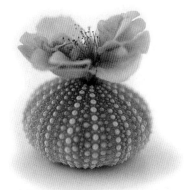

The most successful treatments for PMS include those that effectively switch off the ovaries, since no working ovaries means no PMS. Estrogen implants work amazingly. But sadly the benefit may not last, since the body adjusts to a new hormonal balance and the natural cycle reimposes itself.

Our experience at the NHAS, and the experience of others who have published their results, show that PMS can be helped with a change of diet, the use of certain nutritional supplements and exercise. These factors can all influence female hormone function, the chemistry of the nervous system, general wellbeing and physical fitness in a more gentle and effective way than the 'best' hormonal treatment. A study carried out by the NHAS looked at the relationship between previous PMS symptoms and current menopausal symptoms. Mental symptoms did seem to show some kind of continuity from PMS to menopause, with some small connection in relation to symptoms such as anxiety, depression, confusion and insomnia.

However, there was little or no link with physical symptoms, such as hot flashes and night sweats, suggesting that symptoms mainly due to estrogen withdrawal are not greatly influenced by a history of PMS. In our experience, diet and lifestyle seem to make a big difference to presence and severity of many women's PMS symptoms, which is good news if you are going through similar mood changes at the time of menopause.

Fluctuating hormone levels may not be the only trigger of menopausal symptoms. The many surveys that we have carried out at the NHAS suggest that dietary and lifestyle factors at this time of life can also play a significant part. Pregnancy and breastfeeding, as well as nutritional imbalances that may have developed over the years as a result of dieting, poor eating habits or malabsorption, often take their toll, leaving many of us in a nutritionally depleted state as we approach menopause.

Menopause also tends to hit most of us at a psychological turning point, when natural fears about aging and what the future may hold start weighing on our minds. You may be overloaded with other problems, such as the ups and downs of life with teenage children, caring for elderly relatives, changes in your relationship if you have one, or perhaps doing a job outside the home for the first time in years. If, on top of all this, you have the menopause to deal with, it's not surprising if you feel below par!

Despite all the changes you may be experiencing, it is important to keep things in perspective. The menopause needn't be the end of life as you once knew it, rather the beginning of a new phase that can be just as exciting and rewarding as your earlier years. As long as you take into account all of your symptoms, there's a lot you can do to make this transition as smooth as possible.

What You Can Do

Over the past 20 years, by far the most popular treatment for menopausal symptoms has been Hormone Replacement Therapy (HRT). However, reports over recent years connecting HRT with an increased risk of breast cancer and heart disease has seen this therapy fall from grace. As a result, many women have tried to come off HRT and found an alternative to controlling their symptoms. After 20 years of helping women through their health problems at the NHAS, I can put my hand on my heart and say with certainty that an effective, scientifically based, natural alternative is available. Published research clearly shows that you can overcome menopausal symptoms, as well as protect yourself against heart disease and osteoporosis in the longer term, without HRT.

The results speak for themselves: our latest audit of 100 women on the NHAS Natural Menopause Program found over 91% weaned themselves off HRT successfully without any significant symptoms. In addition, 66% of these women were completely, or almost completely, symptom-free within five and a half months of starting the program. A further 22% experienced some improvement in symptoms. The non-HRT users in particular experienced a dramatic reduction in the severity of their symptoms, with most going from severe to only mild symptoms during the course of the program. More than half the women also said their home life had improved and they were more productive at work.

Getting Started

Throughout the book, I will reveal the secrets to our success, allowing you to devise your own program to help you through the menopausal years. Key areas we will focus on include:

- The truth about HRT and how to come off it
- Replenishing estrogen levels naturally
- Relaxation, which can dramatically reduce hot flashes and help you feel more in control
- Stress reduction and relaxation techniques
- Regular exercise and improving your fitness
- Building up your bones and muscle strength
- Protecting your heart and cholesterol levels
- Sharpening your brain to improve memory
- Rekindling your libido and self-esteem
- Regaining your zest and vitality for life
- Correcting any nutritional deficiencies
- Following a diet rich in phytestrogens
- Benefits of nutritional supplements, including phytestrogen-based, hormone-moderating supplements that are scientifically tested

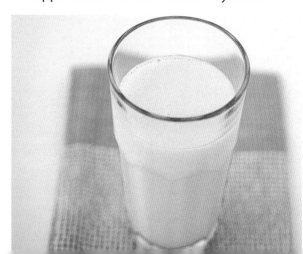

The Symptoms

Menopausal symptoms can be divided into three main groups:

1. Estrogen Withdrawal Symptoms

- hot flashes
- night sweats
- urinary symptoms
- loss of libido
- vaginal dryness
- difficulties with intercourse

2. Other Physical Symptoms

- aches and pains
- migraines and headaches
- fatigue
- constipation
- irritable bowel syndrome

3. Mental Symptoms

- anxiety and panic attacks
- irritability
- mood swings
- depression
- confusion and/or memory loss

Test Yourself

If your periods start to become erratic, or you haven't had one for several months, this could be the start of your menopause. To find out, you can ask your doctor to do a test, or you can do one yourself with your Beat Menopause Naturally home testing kit.

The test examines levels of Follicle Stimulating Hormone (FSH) in your urine. Before menopause, the normal range for FSH levels is up to eight units per litre. As you go into menopause, your levels of FSH may go as high as 100 units per litre.

It usually remains at a high level for two years, or until your brain gets the message that your ovaries are no longer producing estrogen. At this point, FSH drops back to pre-menopausal levels.

Throughout the childbearing years your hormone levels fluctuate during the menstrual cycle, which includes the levels of FSH. For this reason you will need to do the menopause home test twice. Do it once and then repeat it one week later.

If your FSH levels are only high on one of the tests then it's likely that you haven't reached the menopause, but if both tests show a high reading then that confirms that you have arrived.

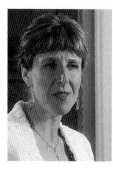

Mairin's Story

Mairin Gallagher had sorted out her PMS with my help 10 years ago. She had stayed in good shape for many years, but she became perimenopausal in her early 40s when she was going through a stressful period. She came back for help as she felt she had lost control.

I had been coasting along nicely for years after sorting out my severe PMS in the early 1990s. I suppose I got complacent along the way, as things were going so well. I didn't really pay much attention to myself as I was too busy dealing with the needs of my family. My teenage daughter was going through a 'wild child' phase and my husband had a nervous breakdown.

I managed to cope with it all, but I was in a bit of a daze one day and I got knocked off my bicycle by a car. It was only then, when I had to take time off from work to recover, that I realized how badly I had let things slip. My periods had become irregular and very heavy, leaving me feeling drained. My mood swings and depression had returned and I was feeling incredibly tired.

I felt like I was losing control and I couldn't work out why my PMS was suddenly back with a vengeance. Maryon had helped me before, so it seemed natural to return for a review consultation. When I got back in touch with Maryon, I didn't realize I was perimenopausal, although with hindsight I should have expected an early menopause because my mother had also started hers in her early 40s.

I made all the changes to my diet that Maryon suggested and changed my supplement regime, which included taking Promensil, and I got back to exercising. I also retrained as a special needs assistant, then eventually decided to go to university to train as a speech therapist. That was such a great achievement, which I would not have even been able to contemplate before.

My periods are much more regular now and the flooding has stopped. I am far less stressed and have coped really well with my daughter's teenage pregnancy and supported her and the rest of the family with lots of new-found energy. I am back in control of my life and I feel much more alive and energetic. I am fully briefed about how to get through perimenopause in good health and much more at peace with myself. I am very grateful to Maryon for her help and advice.

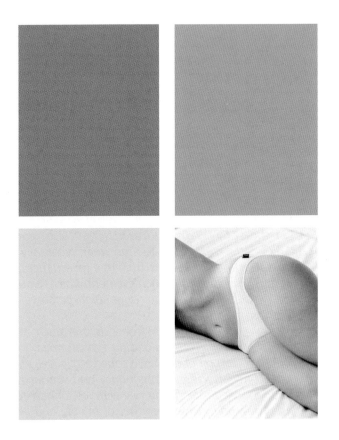

notes

39

"I'm happier, sleeping well and more contented.
I don't lose my memory any more, I'm very on the ball and young
again in my mind."

Sharyn McLaughlin

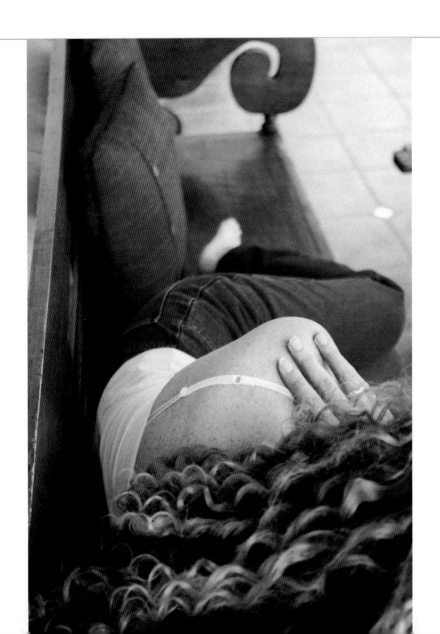

you are not alone

Like many things in life, menopause has its pros and cons. It brings with it a 'minestrone' of emotions. While most women are delighted that they no longer have a monthly period, many of the other signs and symptoms of menopause are usually not so welcome. Many of us are conditioned to believe that the menopause signals the start of old age and we may possibly feel threatened that our partner will become more interested in a younger woman.

Perhaps because we often naturally put the needs of others before our own, we don't make time to exercise or look after ourselves properly. The changes to our appearance and our waistline occur so gradually that it's not until one day when we glance in the mirror that we realize just how far south we have travelled!

Although you may have lived in dread of certain aspects of menopause, one thing I have noticed our patients have in common is that after going through our program they regain their zest for life, their physical shape and self-esteem and often end up feeling better about themselves than they can ever remember.

At the NHAS, we undertook a survey of 500 women going through menopause to see how they really felt about this phase in their lives.

Menopause Survey (2002)

In 2002, we surveyed 500 women who had recently gone through menopause to determine the most common symptoms. It was interesting to note that there are many other symptoms - apart from hot flashes, night sweats, insomnia and dry vagina - that cause major problems. It was also a revelation to discover that nearly twice as many women on HRT lost their libido compared with those who had not chosen the hormone option.

Attitudes

Delighted periods had stopped	80%
Looked forward to more leisure time	45%
Afraid of their physical appearance	40%
Felt menopause signaled the start of old age	37%
Pleased to grow old gracefully	33%
Dreaded their menopause	17%
Thought partner would prefer a younger woman	17%

Physical Symptoms

	% Who Suffer
Hot flashes	74%
Night sweats	70%
Disturbed sleep	73%
Poor concentration and memory	72%
Reduced libido	65%
Aches and pains	64%
Vaginal dryness	53%

Other Complaints

Headaches	47%
Constipation	42%
Bad breath	26%

Mental Symptoms

Anxiety	59%
Confusion	58%
Loss of confidence	55%
Irritability	54%
Depression	49%

Menopause Survey (2003)

In January 2003, the NHAS surveyed another 500 women going through menopause. The most common menopausal symptoms were:

Disturbed sleep pattern	84%
Hot flashes	83%
Night sweats	80%
Poor concentration and memory	72%
Aches and pains	72%
Reduced libido	64%
Depression	64%
Headaches	60%
Vaginal dryness	59%

Sixty per cent of the women had visited their doctor for advice on treatment of menopause-related problems. Only 17% of these women were offered an alternative to HRT.

Many women had sought alternatives and many had tried two or three different alternatives. The popularity of these measures and the self-assessed degree to which they provided a benefit are presented in the following table:

	Number Helped	Total %	No Help	Some Help	Very Helpful
Multivitamins	1202	61%	39%	53%	8%
Vitamin E	842	65%	35%	55%	10%
Minerals	691	64%	36%	55%	9%
Isoflavone	397	79%	21%	59%	20%
Homeopathy	373	62%	38%	52%	10%
Acupuncture	117	59%	41%	40%	19%
Ginseng	366	52%	48%	44%	8%
Don Quai	274	61%	39%	50%	11%
Reflexology	191	67%	33%	55%	12%
Yoga	331	73%	27%	55%	18%

Other Options

Women were also asked what further changes they would be willing to make to try to control their symptoms. The results are presented in the following table:

Treatments Women Would be Willing to Try to Control Menopausal Symptoms

	Very Willing	Moderately Willing	Not Willing
Modify diet	56%	42%	2%
Use natural products	77%	22%	1%
Relaxation therapy	59%	36%	5%
Physical exercise	54%	42%	4%
Take HRT	14%	36%	50%
Take other medication	13%	50%	37%

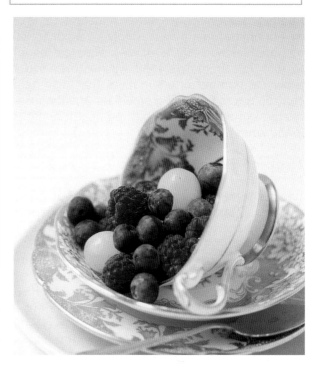

Natural Approach

Sixty seven per cent of women surveyed preferred to manage their menopause naturally. The most popular approach was to use a natural product. Relaxation therapy, increased physical exercise and diet modification were very acceptable to over 50% of women. In particular, 79% of women self-reported that isoflavone-rich supplements were of some help or very helpful.

It would appear from this survey that an increasing number of women are either reluctant to take HRT or are becoming increasingly aware of actual or potential side-effects of HRT. They are eager to look for alternatives and willing to consider a diverse number of alternatives that may help control not only their immediate menopause-related symptoms, but also bring health benefits in the longer term.

Changing Moods

Two separate recent studies indicate that many women approaching menopause should expect to experience their first bout of depression as a matter of course. I found this an alarming finding and one I cannot agree with, as I am very aware that symptoms of depression can be induced by low levels of essential nutrients, many of which are in short supply as we age. In my experience, when our needs are met and nutrient levels are restored to an optimum range, symptoms of depression can significantly improve. Medical literature confirms that psychological symptoms including depression can result from a deficiency in important nutrients, including magnesium, essential fatty acids, B vitamins, zinc and Vitamin C. So our nutritional state very often governs the color of the lenses through which we see life.

In the early days at the NHAS, we began helping women with PMS and treated tens of thousands of women with PMS all over the world. In the course of our work, we measured nutrient levels of many of these women. In three separate published studies, we found that 50%-80% of these women had low levels of magnesium in their blood. Many also had very low levels of B vitamins, iron, zinc and essential fatty acids.

This is also highly relevant to normal hormone function for the mineral magnesium, as well as those other nutrients that were found to be in short supply. Magnesium is necessary for normal brain chemistry, as well as hormonal harmony and the optimum function of our muscles. The brain chemistry is a bit like the conductor in an orchestra, so when it's not functioning too well, it will affect many other departments of the body.

As part of our successful program, we teach people how to get their nutrient levels back into the desired range by educating them about foods that are rich in these important nutrients so they can make their diet more nutrient-dense. We also recommend specific supplements that have been through properly conducted clinical trials, which act as a nutritional prop in the short-term, especially when diets have been inadequate.

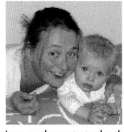

Zoe's Story

Zoe Howes went through an early menopause in her 20s after having chemotherapy.

I was devastated when I discovered I was going through an early menopause. And if that wasn't enough, I was told my ovaries were shrivelled and I would never be able to have a baby. I felt abnormal and had a strong feeling that no man would ever want me.

My periods became erratic and I suffered awful mood swings. I was horrible - really bad-tempered, grouchy and snappy. I would go months without a period, then have two heavy ones, one after the other. I also started to get night sweats and hot flashes. My body felt like it was going mad.

I heard about the NHAS program and decided to try it. After just three months, I had managed to get my symptoms under control, although it was 18 months before my periods returned.

I lost weight and I felt and looked utterly different. People could hardly believe I was the same person. I met a wonderful man and managed to conceive. We're now married with a baby who is just over one year old. I can't describe how much difference the program has made to my life!

notes

"It worked wonders for me.

Within a couple of weeks I was feeling totally new again!"

Marva Morrison

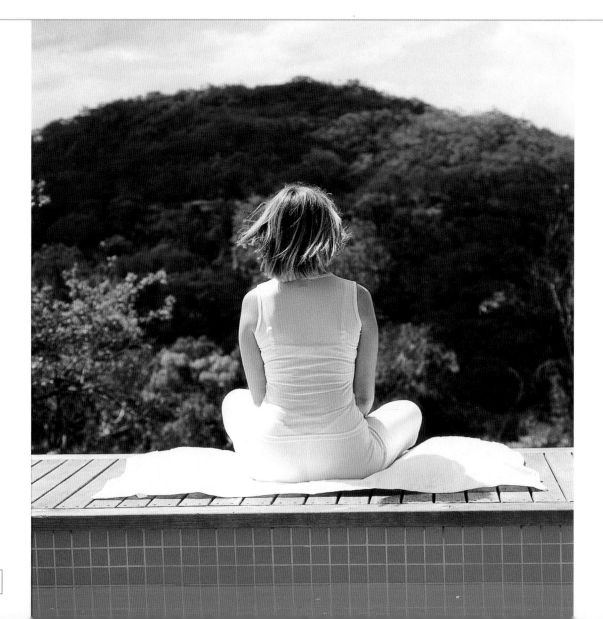

alleviating the symptoms

We all respond differently to menopause. Some women sail through and honestly wonder what all the fuss was about. But for many others, the hormonal swings bring about body changes and unwanted symptoms that can disrupt their lives and result in utter misery.

Constant hot flashes during the day and sweats at night can leave you exhausted, disoriented and despondent. Vaginal dryness and reduced libido can wreck your sex life, while headaches, chronic insomnia and 'fuzzy headedness' can make you wonder if life will ever be the same again.

The good news is that these are menopausal moments, which this book can help you overcome with simple diet and lifestyle adjustments. The only side-effect will be that you feel more like your old self, or in many cases a whole lot better!

So let's look more closely at what causes these symptoms and how you can help yourself in the short-term. As you go through the program, many of the symptoms will crop up again and again. You will learn more about coping with them in the long-term. Some symptoms are interrelated, so you may find that as you treat one symptom, others may also improve.

I Feel So Hot

"I'm having a flash" is a familiar midlife cry. Flashes and sweats can be severely debilitating. No one knows for sure what causes them, but it's thought that a lack of estrogen may affect the action of the hypothalamus, the region of the brain that controls body temperature.

You may be lucky enough to escape hot flashes. However, more than 80% of women are thought to be affected by flashes at some point. They can often start long before you stop menstruating and can continue for several years afterwards.

The frequency, duration and intensity of hot flashes vary from one person to another. You could get several a day, or be plagued constantly day and night. They can last from a few seconds to around five minutes, with four minutes being the average. As well as the sudden rush of heat, you may experience a racing heart, dizziness, anxiety and irritability.

Night sweats are severe hot flashes. You can wake up simply drenched in sweat. You may even have to change your pajamas and your sheets.

If you repeatedly wake up this way, night after night, exhaustion will soon set in. Physical contact with your partner can also trigger a flash, which often causes relationship problems as feelings of rejection set in.

Help Yourself

• Don't be embarrassed by a flash.

• The moment you feel a flash coming on, stop what you're doing. Take several slow, deep breaths and try to relax. This helps reduce the severity of the attack.

• If possible, drink a glass of cold water and sit still until it passes.

• Wear layers of thin clothes that you can easily strip off when you feel yourself getting hot. Clothes made of natural fibres, such as cotton, help your skin breathe.

• Keep your bedroom cool at night and keep a fan, wet wipes and a cold drink by your bed. Use cotton sheets, pillowcases and pajamas.

• Eat little, regular meals. The heat generated by the process of digesting a large meal can sometimes bring on a flash.

• Exercise regularly.

• Quit smoking. Research shows it increases the risk of flashing.

• Include plenty of phytoeostrogen in your diet.

• Try scientifically based supplements.

Did You Know?

The hot surges that can occur in your body are the result of the brain trying to kick-start the ovaries back into function.

Ovarian function does not decline in a straight line, which means that estrogen levels and flashes can rise and fall at different times.

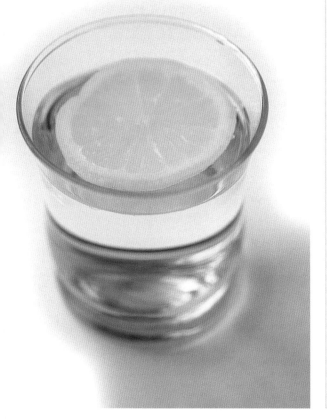

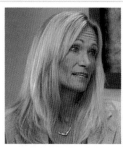

Donna Lothian

Donna is a Nurse Practitioner from Canada.

My hot flashes came on slowly, but before very long they just escalated. I was awake four or five times during the night and I couldn't get back to sleep after I'd had a night sweat. It was impossible to cuddle up with my husband. I had to push him away, as physical contact made the flashes worse. The lack of sleep made it very difficult to function during the day and cope with my job as a nurse. I became moody and got irritable with clients. I got so desperate that I asked my doctor to prescribe HRT, but he didn't want me to go on it and suggested I just go it alone.

I didn't really know where to start at first. I tried taking Black Cohosh, but then I read that it could cause liver damage. I changed my diet by cutting out caffeine, alcohol and spicy food, all of which seemed to make the symptoms worse.

Then I started taking Promensil. After about two months, I noticed big changes. The hot flashes and night sweats dramatically reduced and I started sleeping through the night. I could cuddle up to my husband again and felt so much better once I was sleeping properly. I am now a much happier person, my family has noticed a big difference in my attitude and my children have commented that I'm not moody and snappy any more. I feel much more like my old self and happy to be managing my menopause naturally.

My Head Aches

Headaches and migraines are common during menopause and may be the result of changing body temperature, tiredness due to hot flashes, sleeplessness or general stress and anxiety. Migraines can be affected by estrogen levels and can get better or worse during menopause.

Help Yourself

- Relaxation techniques may help.

- Regular exercise is a must.

- Complementary therapies, such as massage and acupuncture, may help ease the pain.

- Eating an oatcake before you go to bed can help keep blood sugar levels balanced. If they drop during the night, you may wake up with a morning headache.

Having Sex Hurts

The vaginal lining becomes thin and dry as the lack of estrogen causes a decrease in the mucus-producing cells and those cells that keep the walls of the vagina robust and elastic. The result is that sex becomes uncomfortable and in some cases painful. A decrease in muscle tone and subsequent blood supply in the urogenital area may also be a factor. The good news is that this is reversible through diet and specialist supplements.

Help Yourself

- Phytestrogen creams, such as Arkopharma Phyto Soy Vaginal Gel, and Omega 7 capsules help alleviate vaginal dryness and discomfort.

- Regular sex can help vaginal lubrication, as can spending plenty of time on foreplay, since it can take longer to become aroused.

- Pelvic floor exercises help keep your vagina healthy and strengthen pelvic muscles.

Work Your Pelvic Muscles

1. Find your vaginal muscles, if necessary, by stopping a flow of urine mid-stream.

2. With your legs slightly apart, draw your buttocks in.

3. At the same time, draw your vagina inwards and upwards. Squeeze and hold for a few seconds. Repeat 10-15 times a day.

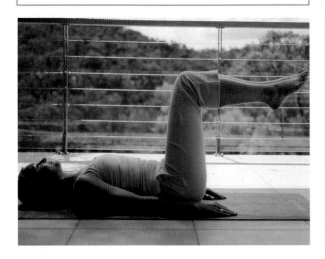

I Keep on Bursting into Tears

Depression, irritability and anxiety are common menopausal symptoms and are probably caused by the hormonal and physical changes you are going through. You may find yourself weeping for no obvious reason, being unable to make up your mind about the smallest things, or panicky at the thought of taking on something that you would normally take in your stride. It is important to realize that these feelings will pass, although it may take some time.

Help Yourself

- Talk about how you feel. Follow a diet rich in phytoestrogen and exercise regularly.

- Try complementary therapies such as yoga.

- Practice formal relaxation techniques such as meditation.

I've Got Terrible Insomnia

Sleepless nights can fast become the norm, so it's important you stop them in their tracks as soon as you can. Usual causes include night sweats, anxiety or having to get up in the night to go to the bathroom. Poor or disturbed sleep can also trigger many other symptoms, such as depression and irritability, so if you start to sleep better, you may also notice an improvement in your moods.

Help Yourself

- Try to include some relaxation and regular exercise in your day.

- Before going to bed, drink a hot soy milk drink or a cup of camomile or valerian tea.

- Listening to soothing music can help you relax and sleep more soundly. Try not to take your worries to bed with you.

- Avoid watching, reading or listening to anything too stimulating in the evening, as it may keep you awake.

- During the night, take the herb valerian to help you get back to sleep until your night sweats are under control.

My Skin is So Dry

Don't worry, you're not alone! Many women start to notice their skin becoming drier around the time of menopause. You may also notice an increase in wrinkles. This is due to the effect that lowered estrogen levels have on collagen, the skin's main structural protein which keeps it firm by supporting and binding its connective tissue. The secret lies in your skincare regime. Try to make sure your skin is well hydrated, both day and night.

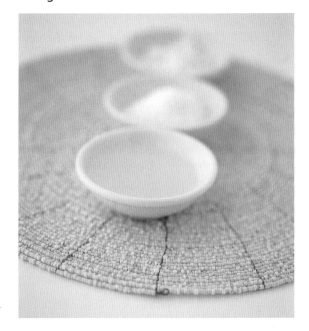

Help Yourself

- Moisturize, moisturize and moisturize again! Look out for Arkopharma Age Minimizing Cream. This is rich in phytestrogen and has a three-fold anti-aging action, boosting the cell renewal process, stimulating collagen synthesis and protecting against free radicals. Recent trials show it can help reduce the depth of wrinkles by up to 48% within four weeks.

- Protect your skin from the sun's damaging rays. Never venture out without first applying sunscreen with an SPF of at least 15 on your face, neck and hands.

- Drink at least eight glasses of water daily to keep your skin hydrated.

- Regularly exfoliate your skin to remove dead skin cells so your moisturizer can more readily penetrate your skin.

- Eat plenty of oily fish, such as salmon and sardines. These are rich in omega-3 fats, which will help keep skin soft and smooth.

notes

Lack of estrogen and essential nutrients at the time of menopause can result in creaking bones and aching joints, especially first thing in the morning. According to our Midlife Survey, women experience far less aches and pains if they meet the health targets of five fruit and vegetables a day, two servings of oily fish a week, regular exercise, no smoking and no more than 14 units of alcohol a week.

Help Yourself

- Each week, eat two to three servings of oily fish, such as salmon, mackerel, herring, sardines or pilchards.

- Most days of the week, exercise to the point of breathlessness for at least 30 minutes. In the morning, try to fit in some stretching exercises to get you going.

- Unlike cod liver oil, which contains high levels of Vitamins A and D and can be harmful in excess, EPA (eicosapantaenoic acid) has been found to help arthritis. The omega-3 fatty acids in EPA create anti-inflammatory prostaglandins that ease the inflammation and pain of swollen joints.

- The supplement Cardiozen, which contains more than 80% of omega-3 fatty acids (of which at least 50% is EPAs), is worth a try. Cardiozen also contains co-enzyme Q10, which is important for muscle energy.

notes

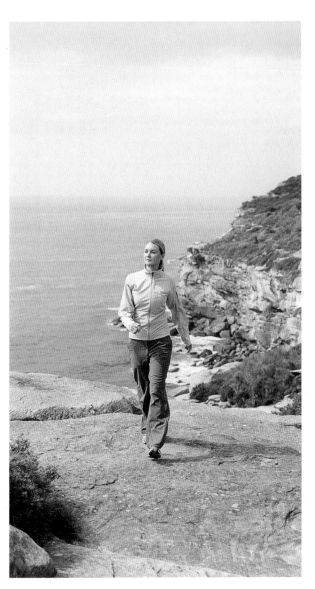

Research File

A small Italian study which was conducted a short time ago suggests that supplementing your diet with polyunsaturated fatty acids (PUFAs) can significantly reduce the number of hot flashes. Under this randomized, double-blind, placebo-controlled, crossover trial, the team in Torino found that PUFA supplements helped 29 women with severe hot flashes enjoy a significant improvement over 24 weeks.

Hot flashes are thought to be partly caused by the brain's response to fluctuating hormone levels. Polyunsaturated fats may help by acting on nerve membranes and neurotransmitters.

Out of 66,500 women attending menopause clinics in Italy, the ones suffering severe hot flashes and night sweats were less active than fellow patients who were more physically active.

The latest data from the Melbourne Women's Midlife Health Project tracked 350 women over eight years. Daily exercisers were less likely to be bothered with hot flashes.

Following a healthy lifestyle and finding time to relax seems to help with hot flashes and night sweats. Eating polyunsaturated fats, swimming or running regularly and cutting down on alcohol and caffeine all seem to help.

"The difference in my symptoms now to before seeing Maryon is quite remarkable."

Eleanor Burns

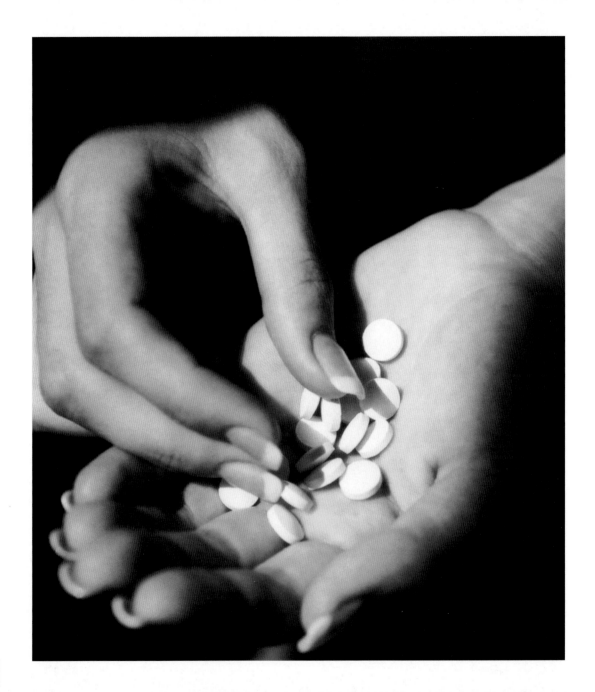

CHAPTER 5

HRT in focus

Until fairly recently, Hormone Replacement Therapy (HRT) was the major breakthrough and considered by many doctors as a treatment for life. It provided the perfect answer to short-term discomforts, such as hot flashes, night sweats, mood swings and a dry vagina. It was also seen as a protector against longer-term risks, such as heart disease and osteoporosis. It seemed there wasn't a symptom that it couldn't help.

Today, following the results of a number of international studies, a different story is beginning to emerge. It now seems, rather than being a cure-all, HRT can increase the risk of breast cancer and may not protect the heart.

As a result, the medical fraternity has had to think again. It has now been recommended that HRT should be prescribed only in the lowest possible dose needed to bring short-term symptoms under control and for the shortest possible time, if at all.

Doctors are advised to review women taking HRT at least annually. If their symptoms persist, they should only re-prescribe the treatment for a maximum of five years, rather than a lifetime. Once symptoms have been quelled, women should be weaned off HRT and encouraged to use an alternative approach.

If you feel you still want to give HRT a try, go through the checklist on the following page to make sure you are a suitable candidate:

- A family history of breast or ovarian cancer

- Undiagnosed vaginal bleeding

- Endometriosis (where the womb lining grows, and subsequently bleeds, outside the womb)

- Severe cardiac, liver or kidney disease

- An impending operation within the next six weeks (an operation can increase the risk of thrombosis)

- Uterine fibroids (HRT can cause heavier bleeding)

- Diabetes (HRT can change blood sugar levels)

- Breast cysts or pain

- A personal or strong family history of thrombosis (blood clots), especially if you are a smoker

HRT may also aggravate:

- Migraines

- Multiple sclerosis

- Epilepsy

- Diabetes

- High blood pressure (occasionally)

- Gallstones

- PMS

Common initial side-effects include:

- Breast tenderness and enlargement

- Premenstrual symptoms, such as mood swings

- Nausea and vomiting

- Possible weight gain

- Breakthrough vaginal bleeding mid-cycle

- Leg cramps

- Enlargement of pre-existing uterine fibroids

- Intolerance of contact lenses

- Patchy increase in skin pigmentation

- Loss of scalp hair

- Increase in body or facial hair

Wean Yourself Off HRT

If you are already taking HRT and want to come off it, take heart. Our latest study of 100 women who had followed our menopausal program revealed that we managed to wean over 91% of women off HRT within five months.

Before coming off HRT, it is vitally important to get yourself established on a scientifically based alternative regime. Details of our successful program for naturally beating menopause appear on the following pages and include an isoflavone-rich diet and a selection of recommended supplements, plus doing some moderate exercise and relaxation. After four to six weeks, the benefits of the program start to kick in and you can begin to reduce your HRT dose accordingly. Research shows that you should wean yourself off HRT gradually, rather than just stopping it, as you can experience fairly severe withdrawal symptoms if you suddenly come off it after taking it for some time.

If you are on a high-dose HRT pill or high-dose patch, ask your GP to prescribe a lower dose for a month or two before stopping HRT completely. Then halve your dose for approximately one month as follows:

- If you are taking pills, break them in half, or take one every second day.

- If you use patches, cut them in half, or use one every second day.

- If you use a nasal spray, use it less, or use it on alternate days.

When you feel the time is right, choose a day to stop taking HRT altogether. If you experience mild flashes during the next couple of months, simply increase the amount of isoflavones in your program and increase your intake of Promensil in the short-term.

Q Bio-identical hormones have been in and out of the menopause headlines recently, but what exactly are they?

A They are made from plant-derived sources of estrogen such as yams and soy products with a molecular structure that is designed to be an exact match with the hormones found in the human body. As such, they are thought to have fewer potential side-effects than synthetic non-bio-identical hormones found in HRT. They also offer women the chance of taking a medication tailor-made to their own specific symptoms. They may well turn out to be a viable alternative to HRT, but as yet there is no scientific evidence to back up their potential benefits and the long-term effects are unknown.

Denise's Story

Denise Pemberton, from Michaelston-y-Fedw in Wales, was suffering with severe migraines.

Following a very stressful period in my life, when we lost three relatives in quick succession, my migraine headaches reached the point of becoming constant. As I was approaching menopause, my GP tried me on HRT, but it made no impression on the symptoms, so after four months I contacted the NHAS for help after reading an article in the newspaper about their work. I made gradual improvement during the first few weeks of the NHAS Program. Within a few months, I felt so much better that I came off HRT. I now only get the occasional mild headache, I have so much more energy and I'm sleeping better. Two symptoms I had suffered for years - swollen ankles and burning eyes - have cleared up completely. I have maintained a good standard of health ever since I started the program. It's very satisfying to know I'm now in control, thanks to the NHAS.

Did You Know?

Women taking HRT should avoid drinking significant amounts of alcohol because it can increase their risk of developing estrogen-positive breast cancer, according to research carried out by Swedish scientists at the Karolinska Institute. It can also be the trigger for hot flashes and night sweats.

notes

Research File

Doubts about the benefits of HRT began in 2003 when part of a large US trial, The Women's Health Initiative, was halted when it was found that combined HRT (the most commonly prescribed form - a mixture of estrogen and progesterone) increased the risk of breast cancer, blood clots, stroke and heart disease.

Next came the UK Million Women Study. The findings, published in the medical journal The Lancet, showed that women taking combined HRT had double the risk of breast cancer. In 2005, more findings from this study showed that when the rates of breast cancer and endometrial cancer are calculated together, the overall risk is highest for women taking combined HRT. This means that around 3 in 100 women taking combined HRT will develop breast or endometrial cancer within a five-year period. This compares with a rate of around 2.5 women per 100 who take estrogen-only HRT or a newer form of HRT called tibolone, and just 1.5 women per 100 who have never taken any form of HRT.

In 2003, the Well-Hart study at the University of California reported that HRT did not in fact slow down the build-up of fatty deposits in arteries (atherosclerosis) for women who already had the condition, as it was once thought to do. The jury is still out on whether HRT may help slow atherosclerosis for women without pre-existing heart disease.

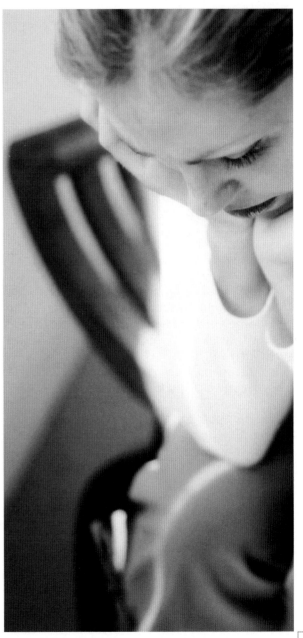

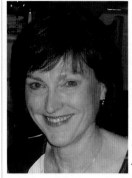

Helen's Story

Helen Benton, a university administrator, lives with her husband Eric and their two daughters, Sally and Marie.

I started getting menopausal symptoms when I was 45. For years, I felt I was only living half a life. I suffered tiredness to the point of collapse, excessive bloating, wind, breast tenderness, pain on ovulation and a gradual loss of interest in sex. I felt totally miserable.

The way I felt affected everything about my life, including my relationships with my family and friends. I used to have such a lot of energy, but found it more and more difficult to cope. That made me feel depressed and reduced me to tears. Eric was sympathetic, but at the same time he was bewildered by the way I had changed. Because I had lost so much self-confidence, I couldn't open up to him, which made him feel shut out.

The girls would say, "Oh, mum's having one of her funny turns again" or "She's in a bad mood again". It was very upsetting. I'd been to the doctor when the symptoms started and he did tests, but said I hadn't reached menopause. So I put up with the symptoms for five years until the doctor finally thought HRT would help me.

I felt very uneasy about it, partly because my mother had breast cancer, although thankfully she had recovered from it. But the doctor said the benefits from HRT far outweighed the risk of breast cancer in my case. He put me on Prempac

C, which is estrogen and progestogen. For the first three months, I felt wonderful, but then some of the symptoms returned. My stomach seemed ten times bigger, my clothes wouldn't fit and I felt frumpy and ugly. I had headaches and migraines and my skin became dry.

I thought my natural periods might have stopped and I wanted to find out. In fact, my periods didn't resume. Instead I had hot flashes about 12 times a day because of the estrogen withdrawal. The heat would start in my stomach and envelop my whole body for several minutes. Afterwards I'd get this cold, clammy feeling, as if someone was walking over my grave. After two months, I thought, "I've had enough. I'm going to take control of my body."

I'd always been interested in self-help remedies. I'd heard of the NHAS and went for a consultation. I began the Natural Menopause Program, which included a change in diet, plus exercise and relaxation. They took me off wheat and caffeine. I was told to eat nuts and pulses and soy-based foods, plus fresh fruit and vegetables three times a day. I was prescribed multi-vitamins and supplements to overcome the hot flashes and guard against osteoporosis. Within a week, I felt a difference. The hot flashes disappeared and I had bags more energy. I felt more positive, much more relaxed and far happier.

Eric is delighted to see the return of the wife he always knew, especially as my libido is returning. I know it's a cliché, but I really do feel like a new woman. I've got my life back and for the first time in years I feel positive about the future.

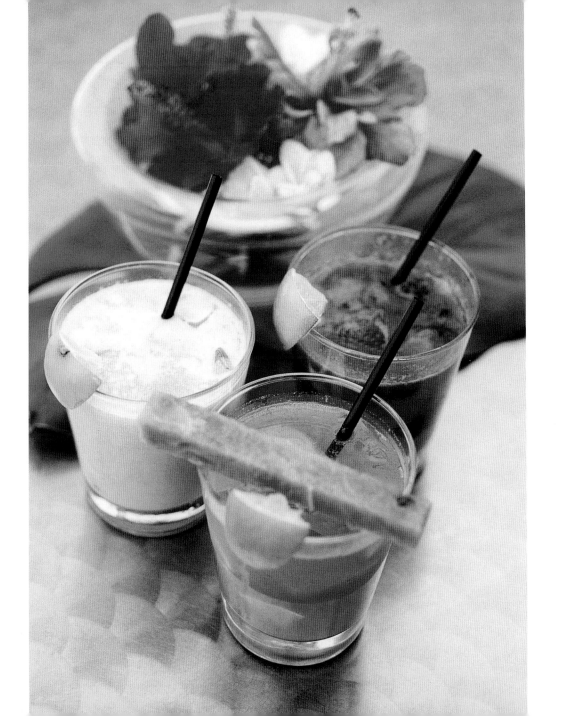

"I feel like I've arrived – it's rather liberating!"

Sue Fisher Hendry

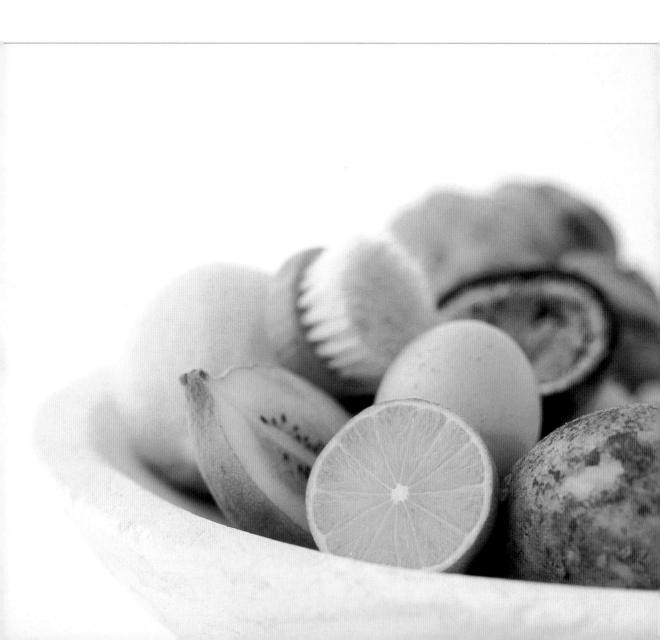

your diet & your hormones

So far we have looked at what menopause is and why it happens. As we have seen, many symptoms can be explained by the natural drop in our estrogen levels at this time. However, this is not always the case, so there must be other underlying causes. It seems our diet and lifestyle and their relationship to our health and wellbeing (or lack of it) may well have a part to play.

Today's diet is very different to that of our Stone Age ancestors. Three million years ago, vegetable matter, including hard seeds and plant fiber such as roots and stems, was the mainstay of our diet, rather than the large amounts of meat protein we consume today. The meat we buy from the butcher or supermarket is also much higher in fat, especially saturated fat, than the wild meat eaten by our ancestors.

Our lifestyle is also very different to what it was even 75 years ago, when three balanced meals with just the occasional in-between snack were the norm. Today, many of us average only one or two balanced meals a day, with around four or five in-between snacks. Life has become much faster, which means we often eat convenience food and pre-prepared meals on the run, rather than the wholesome, home-cooked foods that were favoured by our grandmothers.

Add to this the fact that we now exercise much less and it's not surprising that we suffer from conditions such as heart disease, cancer, diabetes and osteoporosis to a far greater degree than people did even a few decades ago. The incidence of conditions such as irritable bowel syndrome, constipation, diarrhea with gas, bad migraines, nervous tension, irritability, insomnia and feelings of aggression and fatigue are also on the rise.

The Midlife Survey

In 2005, we conducted an online survey of more than 1,200 women between the ages of 35 and 64 to assess their health prospects for midlife. We found that important lifestyle factors, such as diet, exercise, alcohol and smoking, seem to be strongly associated with mental and physical health problems.

The targets needed for a healthy lifestyle that are considered achievable (ie. two portions of fish a week, at least one of which is oily, five portions of fruit and veg a day, exercise at least five times a week, no more than 14 units of alcohol a week and not smoking) are being achieved by less than 25% of people in this age group.

On a more positive note, 75% of the women said they were willing to modify their diet, 77% were willing to do more exercise, 55% would consider taking supplements and 40% were willing to incorporate relaxation into their timetable.

Eighty three per cent had never heard of phytoestrogen. This lack of education was the main underlying cause for decreased feelings of wellbeing. In our experience, once this education is provided, long-term health prospects quickly improve.

The Midlife Survey clearly demonstrated that those women achieving four or five of the healthy targets had better general health, far more energy, fewer aches and pains and good levels of libido compared with those who were meeting fewer targets. The underlying message is that you don't have to make radical lifestyle or diet changes to improve your quality of life and to overcome the various symptoms of menopause.

Other results of the Midlife Survey included:

- 48% admitted to not feeling as healthy as they used to, with only 25% doing adequate exercise.

- Of the smokers, 17% smoked more than 10 cigarettes a day and 8% smoked less than 10 cigarettes a day.

- 25% ate five portions of fruits and vegetables a day.

- 43% ate fish twice or more a week.

- 43% regarded themselves as unfit.

Hormones in the Balance

What we eat influences our health and hormone function. In particular, research shows that hormonal balance can be affected by the amount of fat and fiber in our diet, as well as by the levels of individual essential nutrients we consume.

Although we still don't fully understand the relative importance of these factors, it is safe to say that they have previously been largely overlooked in the treatment of menopause. However, I believe they will become much more important, perhaps to a point where dietary changes are acknowledged as a real alternative to HRT for the control of estrogen-withdrawal symptoms. A change of diet may also help lower the risk of heart disease, as well as hormone-related cancers of the breast and womb.

The Fat / Fiber Conundrum

Scientific interest in the effect of dietary fat on our health originally arose because of its strong links with both heart disease and breast cancer. Research shows that women in countries where diets are high in fat, especially the saturated fat found mainly in animal products, have a high rate of breast cancer. We don't yet know for certain if reducing animal fat intake will reduce the rate of breast cancer, but we do know that the fat and fiber content of our diet can alter hormone function and thus possibly increase the risk of breast disease.

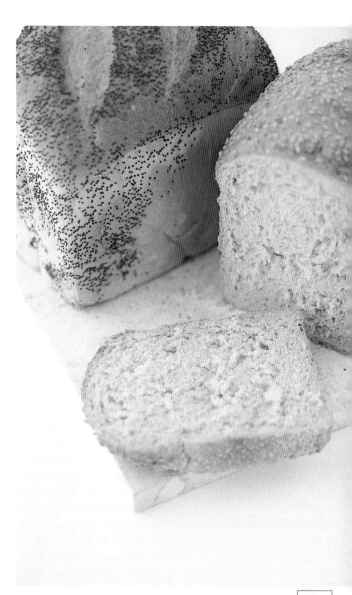

Most studies have shown that:

- A diet high in animal fat and low in fiber is associated with relatively high levels of circulating estrogen.

- Dietary fiber speeds up the rate at which estrogen leaves the body.

- In pre-menopausal women, changing to a low-fat, high-fiber diet can (but does not always) lower circulating estrogen levels.

- Vegetarians and people who are not over-weight tend to have higher blood levels of the hormone-modifying protein Sex Hormone Binding Globulin (SHBG), which helps keep hormones balanced. Severe constipation is associated with a high level of estrogen which can lead to menstrual irregularities.

- Antibiotics can reduce the body's natural recycling of estrogen by killing off friendly bacteria in the intestines.

It's not completely clear what all this means, but it suggests that any extremes of diet and bowel function could be associated with extreme levels of hormones, especially estrogen. It may be that Western women who have followed high-fat, low-fiber diets are much more likely to experience menopausal symptoms due to estrogen withdrawal because their bodies are used to a relatively high level of circulating estrogen. As a result, they don't tolerate the natural drop in estrogen when they reach menopause as well as women who have low levels of circulating estrogen consistently through out their life.

In theory, this means that making a dramatic change from your current diet to a low-fat, high-fiber diet could aggravate symptoms of estrogen withdrawal in some women, although the effect is likely to be offset by the fact that their diet is healthier, which in turn has a positive effect on hormone function. If you do change your diet, it makes sense to do so gradually. For example, don't suddenly go from being a meat-eater to following a weight-loss vegan diet.

Many nutrients are essential for producing hormones and letting them do their job properly. Although nutritional deficiencies have to be severe before they have a profound effect on hormone function, a combination of deficiencies have a subtle adverse effect over the years.

You may think that nutritional deficiencies are rare in countries like America, Australia and the UK. However, authoritative government surveys in these countries indicate that a substantial number of women of childbearing age have a poor intake of a number of nutrients, so there is no room for nutritional complacency.

Our NHAS surveys suggest that many women are not getting enough essential nutrients. For example, 50% - 80% of women with PMS have low red cell magnesium, while B vitamins, zinc, iron and essential fatty acids are also in significantly short supply.

Let's look at some of the more important nutrients and their function:

Iron

The main function of iron is to produce the oxygen-carrying blood pigment, hemoglobin. Your muscles and brain also need iron. Low levels of iron can lead to brittle and split nails, hair loss, fatigue and anemia. Around 4% of women of childbearing age are anemic, but it has to be severe for periods to stop. An additional 10% of menstruating women suffer from a mild lack of iron, causing fatigue. This can also be a problem for perimenopausal women.

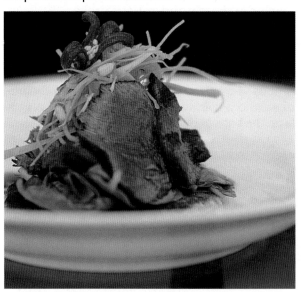

B Vitamins

B vitamins are involved in energy release from food and are vital for a healthy nervous system. A severe deficiency in Vitamins B12 and B3, which is rare, can cause periods to stop or become irregular.

A lack of Vitamin B12, which is found only in red meat, can occur in long-standing strict vegans and in older people who lose the ability to absorb this vitamin. Symptoms include weight loss, fatigue, tingling in the feet and loss of balance.

A lack of Vitamin B3 (nicotinic acid or niacinamide) usually only develops in heavy drinkers, those on very poor, low-protein diets or those with serious digestive problems. Symptoms include depression, dairrhea and a red, scaly rash on the face, the back of the hands or other areas exposed to light. In malnourished women who are deficient in Vitamin B3, menstrual irregularities are common and these may be a problem in perimenopausal women who drink heavily.

Vitamin B6 is often linked with PMS and a mild deficiency is surprisingly common. A deficiency of Vitamin B6, as well as Vitamin B1 (thiamine), is common in both men and women with anxiety and depression. Deficiency in Vitamin B1, however, is not associated with any menstrual disturbance.

Vitamin B6 is involved in the response of tissues to estrogen and seems to be needed by the part of a cell's surface that interacts with estrogen. So increased amounts of Vitamin B6 may be necessary if you take relatively large amounts of estrogen, such as the oral contraceptive pill. HRT seems to have a much less disturbing effect in this respect.

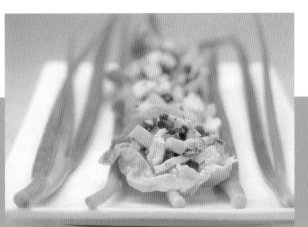
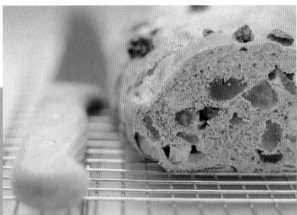

Scientists discovered long ago that a Vitamin E deficiency in pregnant rats caused them to miscarry. In fact, the chemical name for Vitamin E is tocopherol, which is Greek for 'childbearing'.

In women with PMS, supplements of Vitamin E have been found to raise estrogen levels, but the response varies considerably with the dose. Unfortunately, its effect on hormone chemistry in perimenopausal and postmenopausal women hasn't been studied. Its effect on hot flashes, however, has been known since 1949.

In one of the first studies, a positive response of over 50% was recorded when high doses were given. Although this trial was not sufficiently scientific to convince today's doctors, this early study included a woman who started to menstruate again 10 months after she had received radiation treatment to destroy her ovaries! So we cannot completely rule out the results of this trial. Again, it would be interesting to know if some menopausal women have a relative lack of Vitamin E. Lower-than-average levels have been associated with a higher-than-average risk of breast cancer, so supplementation might help some women, perhaps those in perimenopause, rather than those who are postmenopausal.

We sometimes use Vitamin E as part of our program at the NHAS. We find Vitamin E is particularly helpful in maintaining good skin quality and texture. Some women insert it into their vagina on the days when they are not using a vaginal gel.

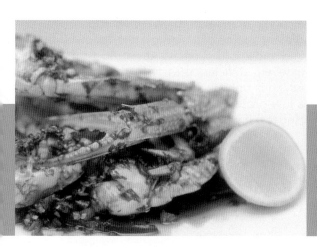

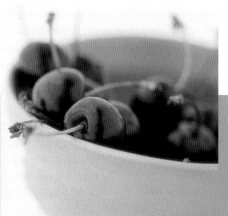

Magnesium

In the past 10 years, magnesium has risen from obscurity to the verge of fame. A cousin of calcium, it is necessary for normal bone, muscle and nerve function. It is also related to potassium and is likewise found mainly inside cells controlling energy functions. Good sources include fresh fruits and vegetables, especially green ones. From dietary assessments, it appears 10%-20% of women of childbearing age consume less than the minimum recommended amount of magnesium.

Magnesium is also involved in hormone function. Experiments have shown that the ovaries need it to respond satisfactorily to the stimulatory effect of the pituitary hormones FSH and LH. A failure by the ovaries to respond is exactly what happens at menopause. Although low levels of magnesium are not the cause of menopause, this mineral often seems to be moderately lacking in women of all ages with premenstrual syndrome. As we know, supplementation can help with PMS, so it wouldn't be too surprising if magnesium had some influence over some menopausal problems.

Good candidates for magnesium supplementation include women experiencing early menopause, erratic menstrual cycles, fatigue, depression or aches and pains. A high-magnesium diet is very nutritious and supplements are harmless enough. The only likely side-effect is dairrhea, which could actually help if you are constipated. No studies have yet looked at the relationship between magnesium and the timing of menopausal symptoms. In our experience, we have seen a variable picture when looking at the results of red-cell magnesium levels, which are known to be low in at least 50% of women with PMS and in some women with menopausal difficulties. Again, however, we cannot blame one nutrient. More comprehensive studies are needed to reach a definite conclusion.

Zinc

Even a mild lack of zinc over time can have a profound effect on sperm and testosterone production in men. As yet, we don't know how important it is for women. Zinc intake in America is fairly close to the minimum recommended amounts and absorption is easily reduced by alcohol, bran and many other foods. The best dietary source of zinc is oysters, followed by beef and most other meats. It would probably take a severe deficiency to upset hormone function, which is only likely in heavy drinkers or those on a low-protein diet. However, see your docor for a zinc test if you think you may be deficient.

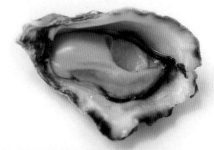

Essential Fatty Acids

As with vitamins and minerals, some fats are essential. These include the polyunsaturates and monounsaturates found in most vegetable oils and oily fish. We've heard a lot about them in relation to heart disease, but the story doesn't end there. First, your body only needs a tiny amount and a deficiency builds up over years, possibly decades, before it takes its toll. A severe deficiency is rare and usually occurs only in premature infants, alcoholics and the malnourished. A mild deficiency can develop in the 'normal' population and this could be a factor in heart disease. Intake of essential fatty acids and blood levels generally fall with increasing age.

On the hormone front, essential fatty acids do something very interesting. They are used in the building of cell walls and, in particular, seem to influence the function of the pieces of cell machinery that are embedded in cell walls, such as hormone receptors. So it is possible that a relative lack of essential fatty acids over many years might modify the way our bodies respond to some hormones at certain levels.

Specialized preparations of essential fatty acids have already been shown to be beneficial in a variety of diverse areas. In our experience, evening primrose oil (omega-6 series) helps women with premenstrual breast tenderness and also assist some adults and children with dry eczema. Fish oils have also made their mark in reducing the pain and inflammation of rheumatoid arthritis. They also help lower elevated levels of some blood fats, but not cholesterol.

According to our Midlife Survey, those regularly consuming a diet rich in omega-3s had fewer aches and pains, less mood swings and less depression, while also having far more energy and an increased libido.

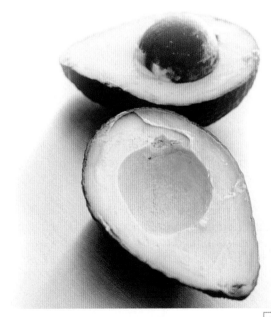

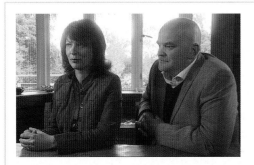

Rosanna's Story

Rosanna Haslam was 36 when she first came to see me. She, and her husband Tim, own a hair salon and have two young children. She was experiencing a whole series of unpleasant symptoms following a hysterectomy a few years before, and felt as if she has lost her grip on life.

At the age of 21, I had two cysts removed from my ovaries, which resulted in me losing most of one ovary. Three years later, I had further surgery to have adhesions removed. In the following few years, I had no further problems and went on to have two children.

A few years after the birth of my second child, I started getting irregular and very heavy periods. This continued for three years and I was treated with D&Cs by my gynecologist. This procedure would help for a couple of months, but then my symptoms would return, and I also began getting extremely tired and irritable. At the age of 30, after four cycles of this, my gynaecologist recommended a hysterectomy. After careful thought, I decided to go ahead, but only agreed to the operation if I was going to be left with my remaining ovary.

I recovered quickly from the operation and had no further problems. About four years later, I started to suffer from severely sore breasts, headaches, depression, irrational mood swings and night sweats. By this time, I felt really desperate, confused and frightened. I didn't feel I could cope any more. I visited my doctor, who was not very sympathetic and prescribed various HRT treatments. Some of these helped with symptoms like the night sweats, but generally made my other symptoms worse and I felt awful.

I was getting into a worse state emotionally and, although many people were sympathetic, no one really seemed to understand what I was going through. While reading a magazine, I saw an article about the NHAS. I called for advice and felt a huge sense of relief when I found that I was talking to someone who really understood how I felt and what

I was going through, so I made an appointment to see Maryon Stewart.

Although the changes I had to make seemed very radical to me, I was driven by desperation and followed the advice to the letter. The results were almost immediate. The symptoms fell away one by one. The following months included regular visits to the NHAS clinic. Each time, I found if I followed the advice, the outcome was positive. If I got complacent and lapsed, or cheated, I really noticed the difference.

I no longer use any HRT and I'm back to feeling full of vitality and life. I cannot express how grateful I am for the help and support I received. I can now run my diet relatively easily and, with my new knowledge of what works for me, I can experiment with new ideas.

I've been told that I look great and I certainly feel good. I've lost weight, got myself back in shape, my cravings for sweets are gone and I feel like I'm back in control. An added bonus is that my libido, which was non-existent, has completely returned and my husband Tim has made it known that he is delighted to have his wife back.

"Rosanna just got her zest for life back and her positive attitude returned with her energy... It was great for myself, our children and our business to have Rose back!"

Tim Haslam

Dandruff: biotin, omega-3 EFAs

Generalized hair loss: iron, Vitamin C

Wrinkles: antioxidants, Vitamins A, C, E, selenium

Eczema: zinc, B vitamins, omega-6 EFAs

Psoriasis: folic acid, zinc, selenium, calcium, omega-3 EFAs

Poor night vision: Vitamin A, zinc

Cracking at corner of eyes: Vitamins B2, B6

Red, scaly skin rash: Vitamin B3

Dry skin: Vitamins A, E

Red, greasy skin at side of nose: Vitamins B2, B6, zinc

Pale complexion: iron, Vitamin B12, folic acid

Cracking, peeling skin on lips: Vitamin B2

Cracking at corner of mouth: iron, Vitamins B2, B6

Red tongue tip: Vitamins B2, B6

Soft, bleeding, spongy gums: Vitamin C

Sore, smooth tongue or recurrent mouth ulcers: iron, folic acid, Vitamins B12, B3

Brittle nails or flattened, upturned nails: iron

are you nutritionally healthy?

Repeated government surveys show that many of us are lacking in nutrients like iron, zinc, calcium, magnesium and some B vitamins. These nutritional deficiencies often underlie our symptoms and affect how we look and feel. Facial acne, greasy skin, cracking at the corners of the mouth, red patches at the side of the nose, acne on the upper arms or thighs, unmanageable hair and split, brittle nails can be our body's way of saying that all is not well. Our body is great at communicating, but the problem is that most of us are not tuned in to interpret the communication. So here is your chance to learn to interpret what your body has been trying to tell you.

The picture on the left and the tables on the following pages outline some of these deficiencies to help you better understand the needs of your body. Be brave and have a close look. You may be surprised how many signs you have suffered.

Realising that you may be short of certain nutrients is the first step. The next step is putting it right. It's not just a question of taking a supplement, but also examining your diet and lifestyle and learning which foods and drinks may interfere with your absorption of good nutrients. Yes, that means that binge eating, too much alcohol and living life in the fast lane take their toll not only on how you feel, but also on your appearance.

What is Your Body Trying to Tell You?

Answer Yes or No for each sign or symptom:

Sign or Symptom	Yes	No	What could it indicate?	Action
Fatigue			Anemia, Vitamin B or magnesium deficiencies, underactive thyroid.	See your doctor for appropriate blood tests (including Vitamin B12 if vegan or vegetarian). Consider taking a good multivitamin and mineral supplement.
Pale appearance			Anemia - iron or folate deficiency. Vitamin B12 deficiency.	See your doctor for appropriate blood tests (including Vitamin B12 if vegan or vegetarian).
Recurrent mouth ulcers			Iron or folate deficiency. Vitamin B12 deficiency.	See your doctor for appropriate blood tests (including Vitamin B12 if vegan or vegetarian). Consider a good multivitamin and iron supplement.
Sore bleeding gums			Vitamin C deficiency.	Take 1000mg Vitamin C with bioflavanoids per day. Visit your dental hygienist.
Excessive peeling and cracking of lips			Vitamin B12 (riboflavin) deficiency.	Consider taking a strong Vitamin B preparation.
Cracking at the corners of the eyes			Vitamin B2 and B6 deficiencies.	Consider taking a good multivitamin and mineral supplement.

Sign or Symptom	Yes	No	What could it indicate?	Action
Cracking at the corners of the mouth			Iron and/or mixed Vitamin B deficiencies. Thrush and eczema.	Multivitamin with iron. See your doctor if it persists.
Red, oily skin at the sides of the nose			Vitamin B2 (riboflavin) and/or Vitamin B6 and/or zinc deficiencies.	Strong B complex supplement and 15mg zinc per day.
Combination skin			Mixed Vitamin B and/or zinc deficiencies.	Strong B complex supplement and 15mg zinc per day.
Persistent dandruff			Biotin and essential fatty acid deficiencies.	Multivitamin, 500mcg biotin and high-strength fish oils. Antifungal, tea-tree or tar-based shampoos.
Eczema			Possible omega-6 essential fatty acid deficiency if excessive dryness.	Evening primrose oil 3,000 mg per day. See your doctor for allergy assessment and infection inspection.
Red, scaly skin			Vitamin B3 (nicotinamide) deficiency in sun-exposed areas.	Strong B complex supplement with 100mg of nicotinamide.
Acne			Possible zinc deficiency.	Zinc supplement 15mg per day (30mg if supervised).
Food cravings			Possible chromium deficiency.	Chromium supplement chart 100 – 200 mcg per day.
Psoriasis			Possible mixed Vitamin B, zinc and essential fatty acid deficiencies.	Strong multivitamin, zinc supplement 15mg and high-strength fish oils. Combine with conventional treatment.

Sign or Symptom	Yes	No	What could it indicate?	Action
Excessively dry skin			Possible mixed deficiency of essential fatty acids, Vitamin A and Vitamin E.	Multivitamin and mineral supplement with evening primrose oil 2,000mg and high-strength fish oil, 400 iu of Vitamin E.
Rough, red, pimply skin on upper arms and/or thighs			Nothing if mild. If severe, mixed vitamin and essential fatty acid deficiencies.	Multivitamin and mineral supplement with evening primrose oil 2,000mg and high-strength fish oil. Better diet.
Depression, low libido, anxiety and PMS			Possible mixed Vitamin B and/or magnesium deficiencies.	Magnesium strong multivitamin and mineral supplement with additional magnesium 150-300mg per day.
Split, brittle, flattened or upturned nails			Iron deficiency.	Iron supplement. See your doctor if it persists.
Ridged nails and white spots on nails			Uncertain significance, possibly iron and zinc deficiencies.	Multivitamin and mineral supplement. Better diet.
Poor hair growth or generalized thinning and loss of hair			Mild iron and Vitamin C deficiencies.	Take iron and multivitamin. supplements and 1,000 mg of Vitamin C. See doctor for specific tests.

Sign or Symptom	Yes	No	What could it indicate?	Action
Loss of sense of taste			Possible zinc deficiencies.	Zinc supplement 15mg per day (30 mg if supervised). See your doctor if it persists.
Poor vision at night or in the dark			Possible Vitamin A (retinol) and/or zinc deficiencies.	Multivitamin and zinc supplement 15mg per day (30mg if supervised). See your doctor if it persists.
Poor appetite			Zinc, iron and/or mixed Vitamin B deficiencies.	Multivitamin and multimineral supplement. See your doctor if you have lost weight.
Wrinkles			Possible lack of antioxidant (Vitamins A, C, E) and the minerals selenium and zinc.	Consider taking a good strong multivitamin and mineral preparation.

Women only

	Yes	No		
Heavy periods with flooding or clots			Iron deficiency.	See your doctor for blood tests, including serum ferritin. Take an iron supplement or a multivitamin with iron.
Painful periods needing painkillers			Possible magnesium deficiency.	Consider taking a magnesium supplement 150-300mg per day, evening primrose oil and fish oil.
Irregular periods			Underweight, low-protein diet and excess alcohol.	Strong multivitamin preparation. Better diet.

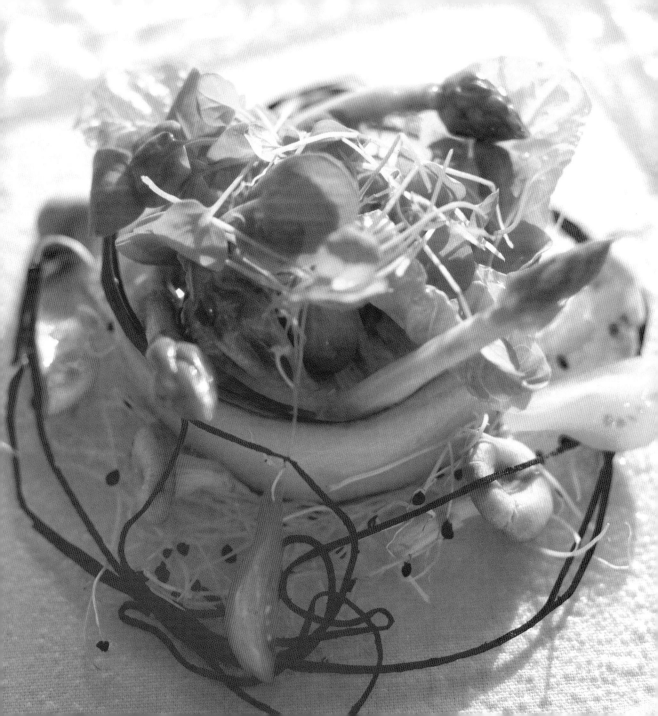

How Did You Score?

If you answered No to all these questions, you're a star! You are in good nutritional shape and don't need to change your diet or take nutritional supplements, unless you particularly want to take a multivitamin and mineral supplement (see page 87) to protect yourself against the potentially harmful effects of our modern environment.

If you answered No to 20-24 questions, you're not doing too badly, but there are some issues you need to address. You should improve your diet by making it more nutrient-dense and also consider taking the recommended supplements according to your particular problems.

If you answered No to less than 20 questions, you obviously need to make some fairly major changes to your diet by following the Naural Menopause Plan and consider taking the supplements that are recommended for your particular deficiencies or physical problems.

Make a note of any possible deficiencies in your Natural Menopause Plan (see page 322). Count your Yes responses and note them down too. You can repeat this test in four months' time and compare your scores to see how much improvement the program has made to your skin, nails and hair.

notes

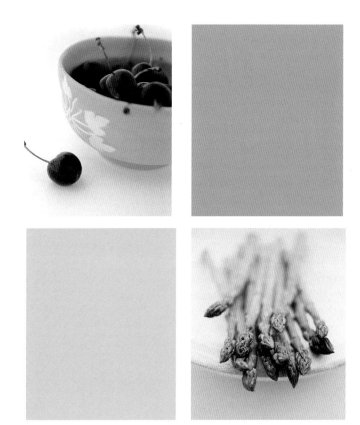

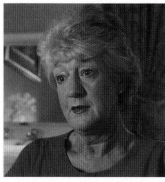

Lynn's Story

Lynn Carr is a 49-year-old Special Needs teacher from Ireland who enrolled in our Telephone Consultation Service. She was perimenopausal and plagued by anxiety attacks and bouts of fatigue.

I had been on HRT following a hysterectomy. When I looked in the mirror, I saw a stranger. My eyes looked blank and listless, my skin color had changed and it looked thinner. I looked white and tired all the time. I felt like I wanted to go to bed, but I was afraid to because I knew I would wake up and not be able to get back to sleep again.

I had gained 13kg on HRT and felt awful about myself. It felt like I had a burning fire in my vagina and I was moody and listless. I was aware that my children were staying away from me at that time of the month. I had low blood pressure and often felt dizzy. I could only describe the feeling inside my head as if my brain was chattering. I was constantly worried about everything and nothing.

I read about the NHAS in a magazine. I immediately called them to arrange a telephone consultation. I was given a series of recommendations to follow and went about implementing them. My first follow-up appointment was six weeks later, by which time all my severe symptoms had become mild. I had so much energy I couldn't believe the difference. Within another four weeks, I could only describe myself as a different person.

You weaned me off the HRT, I lost weight, my vagina feels normal and my libido is back. Everyone comments on how great I look and I certainly feel it.

"I've got my life back and for the first time in years
I feel positive about the future."

Helen Benton

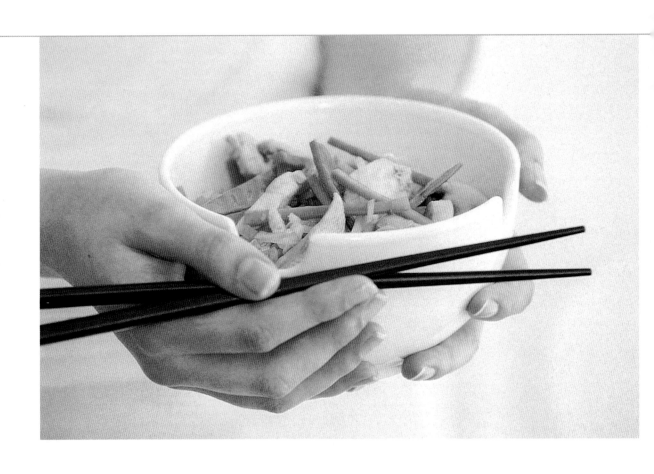

the power of phytoestrogen

You don't want to take HRT, but your symptoms are getting you down. So what can you do? Our successful Natural Menopause Program provides a simple answer. As well as helping restore nutrients into an optimum range, which has a normalising effect on brain chemistry and hormones, the program is also designed to provide regular amounts of phytoestrogen, little and often throughout the day, to fool the brain into believing there is a significant amount of estrogen circulating in the system.

Phytoestrogens are plant chemicals that are similar in structure to human estrogen. They have been hailed by many as the natural alternative to HRT.

Although they are only about 1/1000th as potent as animal-based estrogen, research shows they can help soothe menopausal symptoms and also protect against heart disease and osteoporosis. They may also help lower your risk of hormone-related cancers and block the uptake of excess estrogen by the cells in your body.

How Do They Work?

A wealth of research in recent years has shown that a regular intake throughout the day of phytoestrogen in the form of isoflavones can play a useful part in a menopause control program in a similar way to HRT. Isoflavones, a type of phytoestrogen derived from soy products and red clover, and lignans, another type of phytoestrogen found in flaxseeds or linseeds, have been found to be particularly effective.

In fact, isoflavones are fast becoming known as great hormone regulators due to their balancing effects on estrogen levels. Here's how they work. When estrogen is in oversupply in the body, as can happen before menopause, isoflavones play musical chairs with estrogen, competing for the receptor sites in cells (receptors are structures found on the surface of cells that allow hormones and other chemicals into cells, rather like a key in a lock). Some of the isoflavones inevitably displace estrogen and, being so much weaker in effect, can help reduce the cancer-promoting effects of the hormone.

On the other hand, as estrogen levels start to drop around the time of menopause and beyond, isoflavones can give your levels a natural boost. Combined with supplements and regular relaxation, this can help ease hot flashes and night sweats, and protect against osteoporosis, memory loss and heart disease in the long-term.

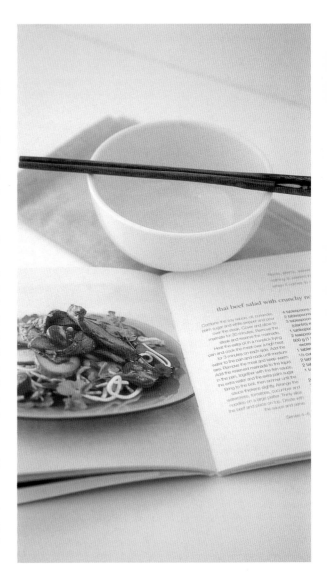

Putting Phytoestrogen into Your Daily Diet

If you're concerned that including isoflavones calls for a radical change of diet, don't worry. There are so many delicious options to choose from that you'll soon find ways to incorporate them into your daily routine. And you don't have to turn vegetarian overnight either.

To alleviate menopausal symptoms, you need to aim for 100mg of isoflavones each day. Working out the exact amount can be tricky because, unlike supplements, foods don't contain summerized amounts. The best way to ensure you get enough is to consume phytoestrogen-rich foods little and often throughout the day as isoflavones appear to leave the body quite quickly. It is thought that isoflavones reach a peak in our blood within six to eight hours of consumption.

As a guide, if you consume a phytoestrogen-rich breakfast, such as Phyto Muesli (see recipes) with soy milk, then have a couple of additional 'phyto fixes', such as a soy and fruit smoothie, or a slice of soy fruit loaf, perhaps in the afternoon and evening, you should start to gain control over your hot flashes and other menopausal symptoms. The list of phytoestrogen-rich foods on the following page shows you the amount of isoflavones in each serve.

The richest food sources of isoflavones are soy products, including soy milk, tofu and soy flour. The most lignan-rich food is flaxseed, sometimes known as linseeds. Foods providing smaller quantities include lentils, chickpeas, mung beans, sunflower, pumpkin and sesame seeds, other beans, green and yellow vegetables (to some extent) and red clover.

Foods rich in phytoestrogen are now readily available from most supermarkets or health food stores, and there are many delicious treats you can whip up yourself in minutes. Soy yogurts are widely available and soy milkshakes make a handy snack. The recipe section of this book includes a delicious fruit loaf made with soy and linseeds, as well as smoothies and fruit shakes, tasty whipped desserts, pancakes and snack bars, all designed to make soy palatable and enjoyable.

Getting your optimum daily intake of 100mg of naturally occurring estrogen is easy once you know which foods to go for and how much phytoestrogen these foods contain.

Phytoestrogen helps to:

- Reduce menopausal hot flashes
- Prevent bone loss, protecting against osteoporosis
- Reduce LDL (the bad cholesterol) and raise HDL (the good cholesterol)
- Unblock clogged arteries
- Normalize blood glucose levels
- Regulate the menstrual cycle
- Help prevent estrogen-dependent cancers (breast, ovarian, prostate)
- Improve cognitive function
- Restore memory

Isoflavone Content of Food

	Isoflavones (mg)
Soy milk (250ml glass)	20
Bowl of Phyto Muesli with soy milk and flaxseeds	30
Tub of whipped soy dessert	20
Soy fruit shake (250ml glass)	20
Slice of soy and linseed fruit loaf	10
Tub of soy yogurt	10
Revival Soy Shake	160
Revival Soy Crispy Bar	160
Tofu (100gm)	25
Soy and linseed bread (1 slice)	11
Phyto Fix bar	10
Soy pancakes (2)	10

Kathy Marynik found Revival products while doing online research and decided to give them a try.

"A number of minor symptoms that I had lived with for years - hot flashes, insomnia, mood swings, lack of energy - disappeared. Plus, I've lost 5 pounds. I can't wait for my next cholesterol check to see if that has decreased too."

Ann's Story

Ann Higgins is a lecturer from Gloucestershire who suffered severely from hot flashes. They were so bad they were making her life miserable.

I had the most horrendous hot flashes, night and day, which ruined my last term as a full-time lecturer and wrecked my life. I'm not exaggerating! During the night, I had up to 12 hot flashes and sweats and probably had twice this number during the day. Sweat would literally run down my face. I had to constantly wash or shower and change my clothes. I felt completely debilitated and low in confidence, since I never knew when a flash or sweat would strike.

Within a week of starting the NHAS program, my energy levels returned, as did my general sense of wellbeing. Within a few months of following the recommended diet, including soy products, taking the recommended supplements and doing my exercise and relaxation, the flashes were non-existent and I was miraculously back to my old self again, and totally cool and calm!

Japanese men, who consume soy products regularly, have plasma levels of isoflavones 100 times higher than their Western counterparts. The health benefits include lower rates of prostate cancer and heart disease.

Can You Overdose on Phytoestrogen?

Asian communities have been consuming substantial amounts of isoflavone-rich food for hundreds of years with no recorded ill-effects. In fact, those consuming a traditional diet have far less heart disease, osteoporosis or estrogen-related cancers like breast, ovarian and prostate cancer. Although studies have used up to 170mg of isoflavones daily for three months and noted positive effects, the long-term effect of high doses has not been studied. The traditional Asian diet delivers 50-100mg of isoflavones per day, so it would seem reasonable not to exceed this dose. This matches the level that has been found to have a therapeutic effect in several clinical trials and therefore seems a safe dosage.

What About Men and Children?

Asian men have consumed significant quantities of isoflavones for centuries without any apparent adverse health effects. In fact, scientists believe that Asian men have a reduced death rate from both prostate cancer and heart disease as a result of their isoflavone-rich diet. Asian children also eat phytoestrogen daily, once again without any adverse health reports. Professor Kenneth Setchell, who has probably conducted more research on isoflavones than any other researcher in the world, believes that the earlier the exposure to phytoestrogen-rich foods, the better.

Fast Facts

- For thousands of years, people in Asia have eaten a diet rich in soy.

- Asian women aged over 45 rarely experience menopausal symptoms, such as hot flashes and night sweats.

- The average daily consumption of isoflavones by the Japanese from their traditional food is 50-100mg.

- Our current daily consumption of isoflavones in the West is less than 3mg.

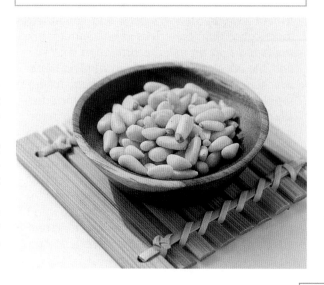

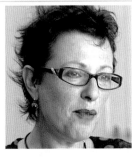

Merle's Story

Merle Shapiro is a jewellery designer from Sydney, Australia. Her symptoms were overshadowing her life and she consulted me when sleep deprivation started to get the better of her and inhibited her daily functioning.

My worst symptoms were the regular and intense hot flashes resulting in an overwhelming sense of lethargy. It turned me into a stranger and even my family said I had such a poor quality of life that it needed to be addressed. I was delighted to find Maryon Stewart's book and comforted to discover that there was a solution to my troubles. I had an initial consultation with her and she gave me a series of recommendations which included making dietary changes, taking supplements, exercise and relaxation. I included soy and roasted flaxseeds in my diet, which made a difference to my symptoms. Even though I'm not really a pill person, I took Promensil and found that the benefits far outweighed any misgivings I had. Within a month, I noticed the intensity of my symptoms had reduced. Over the next month, the flashes almost completely disappeared and I got my energy back. I went from having no real quality of life to feeling absolutely excellent!

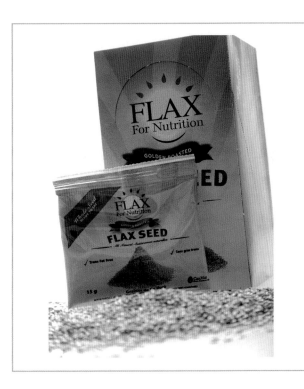

Did You Know?

Until recently the Japanese language did not include the term 'hot flash', largely because Japanese women, who consume a diet rich in phytoestrogens, hardly experience any adverse symptoms at the time of the menopause unless they have switched to a Western diet.

Flax for Nutrition

Rich in omega-3 esssential fats, dietary fiber and lignans, Golden Roasted Flax Seeds by Flax for Nutrition are the perfect way to add naturally occurring estrogen in the form of lignans to your everyday diet. Although the amount varies, there is approximately 30mg of lignans in a tablespoon of roasted flaxseeds.

Since these seeds are roasted, they are much easier to chew than raw flax and they've got a lovely crunchy, nutty flavour. They are also packed in handy, small packets which are ideal for popping in your handbag, so you can have them on hand wherever you are. Flax for Nutrition also produce a range of Milled Flaxseeds that are mixed with apple, cinnamon and blueberries. These can be sprinkled over cereal, salads and chopped fruit.

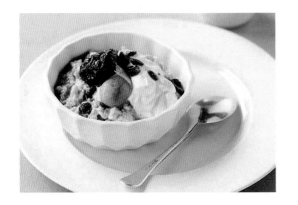

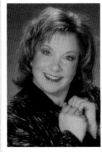

Laurie Campbell

Laurie is a busy 49-year-old woman who works in the administration field with both a full-time and part-time job in Regina, Canada.

My menopause symptoms began shortly after a partial hysterectomy I had when I was 45. I had night sweats that severely disrupted my sleep, leaving me exhausted and with brain fog. I also had a high cholesterol level.

I didn't want to take HRT and preferred to make changes to my diet in order to control my symptoms. Reducing caffeine helped and in addition, I began including roasted flax daily into my diet. Within a few months my flashes diminished and my quality and quantity of sleep improved. From follow-up blood tests a few months later I discovered that my cholesterol levels had returned to normal for the first time in three years. In addition, I noticed that my hair became healthier looking, my skin got back its old glow and I had much more energy.

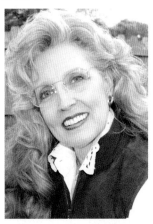

Suzanne's story

Like a large majority of women her age, Suzanne Tabor was experiencing severe discomfort with her symptoms of menopause.

At 50 I was a wreck! 50 is a 'good number' unless it represents the number of hot flashes you're having each night, the number of steps it takes you to wear out, or the dress size you fear may be yours. This is not much of an exaggeration for the condition I felt my life was in. I thought after I raised the kids I would be kicking up my heels. I needed some kind of relief, my family thought that too, trust me.

On the advice of my son who is a medical student, I started trying various forms of soy, but found it hard to consume enough, and found its chalky taste unpleasant. Then I started taking Revival Soy products. Within days I started to feel better. I suddenly had more energy and my menopausal symptoms had almost vanished in four weeks.

Six servings of soy milk a day is what you need to get maximum benefit from soy isoflavones but this may not appeal when you find out that this amount of soy milk can contain up to 24g of fat as well as loads of calories. Also you may be one of those women who cannot stomach the taste of soy.

Enter Revival Soy 'Soy without the Soy Taste'. Just one Revival Soy bar or Shake contains the same amount of isoflavones as six glasses of typical soy milk but without the soy taste and up to 90% less fat. What's more Revival Soy is a' medical-grade' soy product meaning it is used in clinical trials at some of the top medical schools and hospitals in the US.

What's In A Bar Or Shake

Each convenient on-the-go Revival Crispy Bar or Shake contains:

- 20g soy protein
- 160mg soy isoflavones (certified and GMO Free)
- 500mg bone-healthy calcium
- 5g soluble fiber
- Trans-free fat

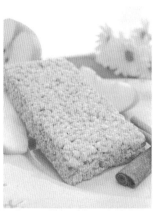

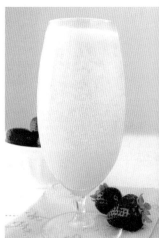

Research File

The following studies, together with a host of others, suggest that phytoestrogen may well be as powerful as HRT in protecting against osteoporosis, heart disease and other unwanted symptoms of menopause.

In 1990, I came across some research by a group of Australian doctors who had put a group of women, who were going through menopause and not taking HRT, on a diet rich in soy products, organic flaxseeds and a herb called red clover, all of which are rich sources of phytoestrogen. They demonstrated it was possible to bring about the same changes in the lining of the vaginal wall in these women as the changes experienced by women taking HRT. This was great news for the 'alternative' camp, proving that phytoestrogen, including soy isoflavones, can reach the same parts of the body as HRT.

According to a study published in The Lancet in 1992, the reason why Japanese women don't seem to experience menopausal symptoms to the same extent as Western women is because their diet contains foods rich in isoflavones, such as soy products.

A few years later, another Australian study showed menopausal women who consumed bread rich in both soy and flaxeeds (another good source of phytoestrogen) showed a 40% reduction in hot flashes and a small increase in bone mass.

Recent research at the University of Insubria in Italy shows that lignan phytoestrogen, in particular Norwegian spruce lignans, act on the physiological estrogen balance and, may offer a natural alternative to help buffer the hormonal fluctuations experienced during the menopause.

According to Mindy Kurzer, Professor of Nutrition at the University of Minnesota, who conducted a formal review of the published clinical studies on soy, there is a positive benefit to consuming soy, despite some negative reports. Professor Kurzer points out the difficulty in comparing one clinical trial with another, given the variables in trials.

In a study carried out in 1998 by Dr Paola Albertuzzi, 104 post-menopausal women took either 72mg of isoflavones or a placebo each day for 12 weeks. The results showed that soy was significantly superior in reducing the number of hot flashes experienced. Women taking soy reduced their hot flashes by 26% after three weeks, 33% by week four and 45% by week 12, compared with a 30% reduction in the hot flashes of the women in the placebo group.

A study of 650 women aged 19 to 86 found post-menopausal women with the highest intake of dietary isoflavones had significantly higher bone mineral density at both spine and hip than those with lowest intakes after adjusting for age, height, weight, years since menopause, smoking, alcohol consumption, HRT usage, and daily calcium intake.

"You're an elder now and you should be proud of it.
It's time to strut your stuff!"

part two

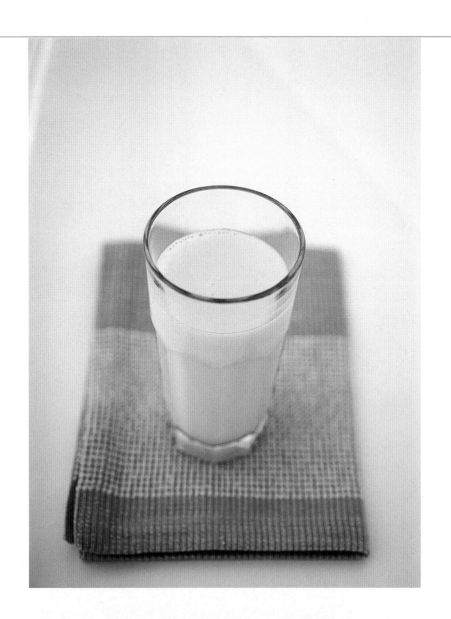

build your bones

Sadly, menopausal moments don't stop with hot flashes and night sweats. Following on from menopause comes another threat to our health. This threat is osteoporosis or brittle bone disease.

Osteoporosis involves a loss of calcium (the mineral in bones) and collagen (the gluey protein that helps strengthen them). As a result, bones become full of gaping holes, rather than the fine, honeycomb texture of normal, healthy bones. Bones lose their ability to absorb shock and eventually become so weak that even a small knock or fall can cause a fracture or break.

So what causes osteoporosis? You may not think of bones as living tissue, but they go through a constant process of renewal during our lives. Until the age of 35, we make as much new bone as we lose, keeping the scales in balance. But from then on, we tend to lose around 1% of our total bone mass each year until we reach menopause. From that point, bone loss accelerates a further 2%-3% per year for up to 10 years.

This is partly due to falling levels of estrogen, as one of the key roles of this important hormone is to maintain bone mass. It is not surprising that our bones become more vulnerable to osteoporosis after menopause. Reduced levels of estrogen are certainly a trigger, but other lifestyle factors are also involved in this process, some of which can be modified to help improve the strength of our bones for life.

113

To assess your risk, start by answering Yes or No to the following questions:

	Yes	No
In your childhood and teens, did you consume a poor diet, low in calcium (especially dairy products)?	☐	☐
Do you regularly consume red meat and dairy products, rather than including vegetarian sources of protein in your diet?	☐	☐
Did you experience an early menopause, spontaneously or following surgery?	☐	☐
Do you have a history of thyroid or other hormonal problems?	☐	☐
Have you been underweight or suffered an eating disorder, such as anorexia or bulimia?	☐	☐
Have you always had a petite build?	☐	☐
Do you smoke 10 or more cigarettes per day?	☐	☐
Have there been times in your life when you regularly drank alcohol to excess (more than the equivalent of 14 glasses of wine per week)?	☐	☐

	Yes	No
Do you only rarely perform formal weight-bearing exercise?	☐	☐
Do you lead a sedentary lifestyle?	☐	☐
Have you had periods of excessive physical activity in your life, eg. an athlete or a ballet dancer?	☐	☐
Have you taken steroid drugs for an extended period of time?	☐	☐
Have you suffered more than one fracture since your menopause?	☐	☐
Has a close relative suffered osteoporosis?	☐	☐
Have you experienced a chronic illness that affected your digestion, kidney and liver function?	☐	☐
Did you ever stop having periods, especially when you were young?	☐	☐

If you answered Yes to just one of these questions, you have a higher than average risk of osteoporosis. If you answered Yes to more than two questions, you need to get going on the Action Plan below as soon as you can. Don't forget to enter your score in the Natural Menopause Plan on page 322.

Action Plan

You can't change your family, but experts now think that the level of bone density you lay down in your lifetime is only 70% due to genetic factors, with the remaining 30% due to lifestyle factors. So even if osteoporosis is in your family, there are still things you can do to protect yourself.

Assess Your Diet

Bone-building is a complex mechanism involving many elements. Calcium is the key, but it's not the only factor. Magnesium, phosphorous, boron and Vitamins C and D are also important. In particular, magnesium helps the body to absorb and use calcium and getting a healthy balance of these two minerals is vital.

Dairy products are very dense sources of calcium, but they contain almost no magnesium. So how do cows grow such large, strong bones after weaning? They eat grass. And this is the clue: any green, leafy vegetable such as watercress, kale, broccoli or cabbage provides the perfect balance of calcium and magnesium. Nuts and seeds also provide balanced amounts of these two minerals.

Get Phyto-rich

Make sure your diet also includes plenty of plant phytoestrogen. Good sources include soy beans, soy products such as tofu and soy milk, flaxseeds and to a lesser degree lentils, chickpeas and mung beans.

Be Sunny

Vitamin D helps your body absorb calcium. The action of sunlight on your skin provides the main source, so it's important to get out in the sunshine. To obtain enough Vitamin D for the health of your bones throughout the year, during the summer months you need to expose your face and arms to the sun without sunscreen for 8-12 minutes per day if you have fair to medium skin, or 45 minutes per day if you have dark skin. If you spend longer in the sun, remember to apply a sunscreen with a sun protection factor of at least SPF 15. Small amounts of Vitamin D can be found in some foods, the main sources being egg yolk and oily fish.

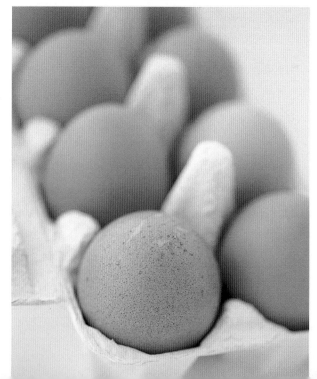

Go for Fats

Research suggests that foods rich in omega-3 and omega-6 essential fatty acids seem to help the absorption of calcium from food. Omega-3s are found in fish oils, oily fish (salmon, mackerel, herring, sardines, pilchards) and some cooking oils, such as rapeseed and flaxseed. Good sources of omega-6s include sunflower and corn oil, almonds, green leafy vegetables, flaxseeds and wholegrain cereals.

Avoid Them If You Can

Try not to have too much animal protein, salt or caffeine, as excessive quantities can reduce your body's ability to absorb and retain calcium. Excessive alcohol is also thought to interfere with calcium metabolism and affect bone-building cells, resulting in loss of bone density.

Exercise Regularly

Exercise plays a vital part in keeping bones healthy. High impact activities that slightly jar the bones are the most beneficial. Running, jogging, brisk walking and lifting weights are all good choices. As you age, gentler alternatives include golf, gardening and dancing. Aim for at least 30-45 minutes of moderate exercise at least four or five times a week.

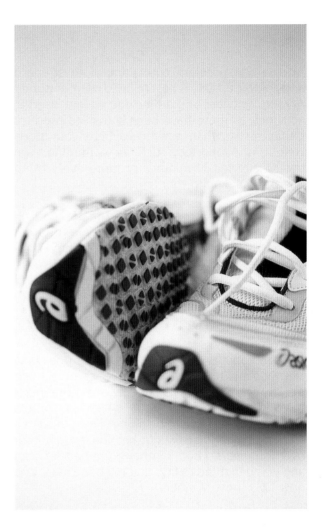

An exercise program combining both strength and aerobic activity is best to build up your bones. Aerobic activities should include weight-bearing activities, as these have been shown to produce better results than activities where your body weight is supported, such as swimming. You should aim for 30 minutes or more every other day, but build up to your target gradually.

Strengthening exercises place a greater load on the bones and make it possible for you to target key body parts, such as the upper spine, hip, wrists and ankles, which are more vulnerable to fractures. You can do these in a gym with weight-training equipment or at home with free weights. Pilates and yoga are also good weight-bearing exercises.

We repeatedly see good production of new bone in patients not taking HRT, but it does take several years to notice the difference on a bone density scan. Nine years ago, my own bone mass measured average for my age, which was quite a shock as I expected it to be higher. Five years later, after doing regular weight-bearing exercise for over four years, I had another bone density scan and was delighted to find that my bone mass was now 17% above average.

Apart from the bone-strengthening benefits, exercise has so many other benefits, especially when performed to your favourite music. Just don't expect miracles overnight. (See page 122).

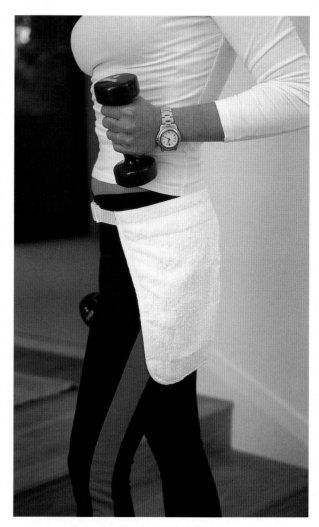

Findings of the NHAS Osteoporosis Survey

We carried out a survey to analyse the link between diet, lifestyle and osteoporosis. The respondents varied in age from 18 to over 80, while the average age was 55.3 years.

The survey revealed that many people are unaware of the nutritional and dietary requirements for preventing osteoporosis, both in terms of optimum calcium intake and types of food required to maintain healthy bones. Nearly 75% of the women were unaware that soy products should be incorporated into an optimum diet to prevent osteoporosis. Over 50% were not fully aware of the importance of calcium in the form of dairy products, while 66% did not do enough exercise to maintain their bone health.

Other results included:

- 5.5% were underweight (less than 51kg)

- 20% had smoked at some time and 17% still did smoke

- 31% said they had a sedentary lifestyle

- Only 28% did at least 3-4 sessions of weight-bearing exercise per week

- 10% had experienced one or more fractures, while 26% had a relative with osteoporosis

- In reply to the question, "Are you afraid of osteoporosis?" 27% said they were considerably afraid, 54% were moderately afraid and 19% were not afraid at all

- 49% consumed 1-2 portions of dairy products per day, while 11% felt it was not essential to consume milk at all to prevent osteoporosis

- 74% felt that soy milk and soy products were not important to prevent osteoporosis

---

What Makes Bones Strong?

- Diet, especially the intake of calcium during the growing years

- Physical activity, particularly weight-bearing exercise

- Hormonal factors, particularly the balance of estrogen

- Genetic factors, which determine the size of bones and muscles

- Optimum levels of nutrients like calcium, magnesium, boron and essential fatty acids

Research File

Japanese women have half the hip fracture rate of Western women, while women in Hong Kong and Singapore suffer even fewer fractures. One explanation could be that Asian women are more active. Japanese women, who traditionally sit on the floor, probably have stronger muscles and bones as a result. But there is more to it than that, as research is beginning to unveil.

Animal studies have compared the effect on bone health of the plant estrogen, genistein and Premarin, a type of HRT. These showed that low-dose genistein can prevent bone loss almost as well as Premarin.

According to Dr John Anderson of the University of North Carolina, genistein's beneficial effects may be due to its weak estrogenic properties. Bone cells, like reproductive cells, have estrogen receptor sites. At menopause, when estrogen levels fall, these bone receptor sites become redundant. However, phytoestrogen may continue the function of natural estrogen, thus minimising bone loss.

Daidzein, another type of isoflavone, also seems to be good news on the bone front. Soy products rich in both genistein and daidzein, the two main types of isoflavones, are officially approved in Europe and Japan for the treatment of osteoporosis as they appear to slow bone loss and stimulate growth of new bone. The same is true for Novogen's supplement Promensil. Researchers are still trying to figure out why soy seems to spare calcium more than animal protein. One theory is that soy protein has low levels of the sulphur that contains amino acids, which cause production of sulfate in urine.

Sulfate prevents calcium from being reabsorbed into the bloodstream, instead being excreted through urine. In addition, most high-protein foods contain phosphorus, which, although reducing the amount of calcium lost in urine, actually increases calcium loss through bowel movements. This may put regular meat-eaters at an even greater disadvantage, since meat contains low levels of calcium.

Professor Kenneth Setchell studied 43 post-menopausal women who consumed 60-70mg of isoflavones per day for 12 weeks. He found that osteoclast (bone-dissolving) activity decreased by 14% and osteoblast (bone-forming) activity increased by 10%. These findings indicate reduced bone loss for women on an isoflavone-rich diet.

Another interesting study by Lee Alekel showed that 80mg of isoflavone-rich soy protein per day for 24 weeks was significantly bone-sparing in the lumbar spine of perimenopausal women.

Another type of isoflavone, formononetin, has been shown to help bone regeneration. A double-blind randomized placebo-controlled trial of Novogen's Promensil isoflavones - providing a daily dose of 26mg biochanin A, 16mg of formononetin, 1mg of genistein and 0.5mg of daidzein for one year - showed that loss of lumbar spine bone mineral content and bone mineral density was significantly lower in women taking the isoflavone supplement compared to those taking the placebo. During menopause, bone density normally reduces by up to 7%-8%, but in those taking the supplement there was a decline of only 3%-4%.

A review of 18 randomized controlled trials, led by the Cochrane Collaboration, found that aerobics, weight-bearing exercises and resistance exercises all help strengthen your spine after menopause. Walking also helps make the hip bones stronger.

The Way Forward

The optimum regime for better bone health should encompass all aspects of this research. We should include calcium in our diet, increase our intake of soy protein, take Promensil and reduce our intake of animal protein.

It appears the 'calcium only' crusade may have backed the wrong horse by treating osteoporosis as a deficiency disease. If it is a deficiency, it must be one of estrogen, rather than calcium. Lower levels of estrogen can also trigger a decline in bone density. This is why regular weight-bearing exercise is so important.

Joanne's Story

Joanne Simms, a mother of two from Toronto, Canada, was diagnosed with early onset or premature osteoporosis.

I went through an early menopause in my early 40s. I had a bone density scan and was shocked to discover a 7% loss of bone mass in one year. I was advised to take long-term medication, but after reading Maryon Stewart's book, Beat Menopause Without HRT, I decided to give myself a year of natural solutions before accepting the drugs as the solution.

I went and saw Maryon, who helped me refine my program. This involved making significant dietary changes, taking nutritional supplements and doing daily weight-bearing exercises.

A year later, my follow-up bone density scan showed almost no further bone loss and the advice this time was 'keep taking the tablets'. I'm hoping that next year's scan will show I have made some new bone. I'm certainly feeling well and much fitter as a result of my new regime.

Upper Spine

1. Lie flat on your back on the floor or on a bed. Press your head backwards and push for a count of five. Release and repeat. Don't hold your breath (counting out loud can help), since this can increase your blood pressure.

2. Lie on your stomach, preferably on a hard surface. Squeeze your shoulder blades together, then try to lift your head and shoulders straight upward a few inches off the floor, without bending your neck backwards. Lower and repeat a few times. Gradually increase the number of repetitions. Keep looking at the floor at all times so your spine remains in a straight line.

3. In a seated position, pull your shoulder blades together and hold briefly. Repeat 10 times.

Hips

1. Standing on one leg, lift your other leg out to the side in a smooth, controlled manner, then lower it back down. Repeat 10-15 times, then swap legs.

2. Ensure you stand upright throughout the movement and don't allow the supporting hip to push out to the side to compensate. This exercise can also be performed while lying on your side with your upper leg traveling in a vertical plane.

3. Alternatively, lie on your back with your knees bent and your legs positioned on the inside of the legs of a chair. Try to push your knees and legs apart (the chair legs will prevent this). Hold for a count of five, then release. Remember not to hold your breath.

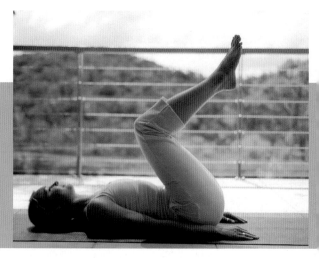

Ankles

1. Stand upright, gently leaning against a chair or bench, and lift your heels off the floor.

2. Check that your ankles do not roll outwards and keep your weight over your big toes.

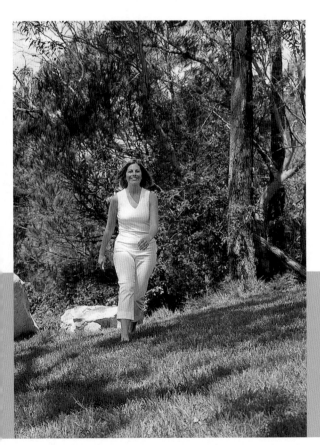

Wrists

1. Stand an arm's length from a wall, arms straight out, with your hands flat on the wall at shoulder height.

2. Slowly bend your elbows, bringing your face and chest closer to the wall, then pushing back out (like doing a push-up against the wall). Repeat 10-15 times.

3. As you become more proficient, you can perform this exercise on the floor on your hands and knees. In this position, you should gradually lower your body towards the floor, keeping your back straight.

"Activity…get it into your everyday lifestyle.
There are three immediate benefits of exercise
and they all begin with the letter 'S'.
There's Suppleness,
keeping our bodies Stronger
and Stamina."

Diana Moran

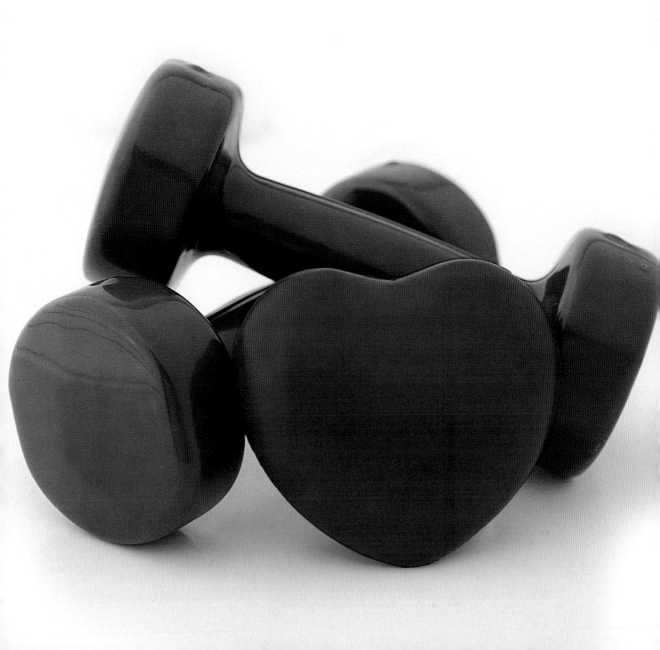

CHAPTER 10

get heart healthy

You may think of heart disease as predominantly a male problem. Indeed, before you reach menopause, your risk is much lower than for men of the same age. Researchers are not sure why this is, but it is thought that estrogen may help protect women during their childbearing years.

However, after menopause, women's risk of heart disease - including atherosclerosis (blocking and hardening of the arteries), high blood pressure, angina, heart attack and stroke - is similar to that of men. After menopause, 30% of women will develop heart disease. So let's look at the reasons why and, more importantly, how heart disease can be prevented.

It seems that menopause brings changes in the level of fats in the blood known as lipids, which determine your cholesterol level. There are two components of cholesterol: high density lipoproteins (HDL), which is associated with a beneficial, cleansing effect in the bloodstream, and low density lipoproteins (LDL), which encourages fat and mineral deposits, known as plaque, to accumulate on the walls of arteries, causing them to narrow and clog up.

In post-menopausal women, as a direct result of estrogen deficiency, LDL cholesterol appears to increase, while HDL decreases. An elevated LDL and total cholesterol level is linked to a higher risk of stroke, heart attack and death.

To assess your risk, start by answering Yes or No to the following questions:

	Yes	No
Do you smoke?	☐	☐
Do you exercise less than 3-4 times a week?	☐	☐
Do you eat a lot of fatty foods, such as hamburgers and red meat?	☐	☐
Are you overweight?	☐	☐
Do you have high blood pressure?	☐	☐
Is your cholesterol count high?	☐	☐
Do you drink more than 14 units of alcohol per week?	☐	☐
Do you eat fish, especially oily fish, less than twice a week?	☐	☐
Do you eat less than five portions of fruits and vegetables a day?	☐	☐

If you answered Yes to more than three questions, you need to switch to a heart-friendly lifestyle as outlined below. Don't forget to make a note of your score in your Natural Menopause Plan on 322.

Action Plan

• It has been known for years that the saturated fats found mainly in animal protein, such as meat, dairy products and eggs, can contribute to atherosclerosis, so you should aim to cut down on fatty foods such as burgers, sausages and pies. But this doesn't mean you need to cut out fat completely. Monounsaturated fats, found in olive oil and rapeseed oil, and polyunsaturated fatty acids, derived from a variety of plants, flaxseeds, fish oils and cold pressed flaxseed oil, can shift the balance towards the good HDL cholesterol, although the degree of protection these ' healthy' oils offer is still under debate.

• Most experts now agree that if you want to reduce your risk of heart disease, you must cut down on saturated animal fats, stick to a modest intake of polyunsaturated fats and maintain your intake of monounsaturated fats.

• Drink alcohol in moderation and make sure you eat at least five portions of fruits and vegetables every day.

• Try to include oily fish, such as salmon, mackerel, herring, sardines and pilchards, in your diet at least twice a week. Research shows that omega-3 fatty acids in these fish can help protect against heart and circulatory disease.

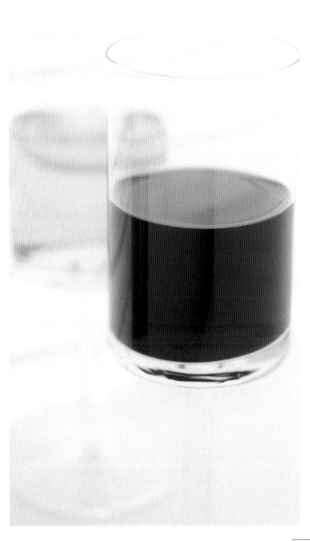

129

Get Moving

Regular aerobic exercise at least five days a week will help keep your heart and circulation in good shape. Aim for 30 minutes a day, but you can divide it up into 15-minute bursts if you prefer. You need to exert yourself enough to feel warm and slightly breathless, but still able to hold a conversation. If you're unfit, start gently by taking regular walks and gradually increase to a level you feel comfortable with.

Give Up Smoking

If you are still puffing away, give up now for the sake of your heart. Smoke-damaged arteries attract fatty deposits that restrict the blood flow to your heart muscle. Smoking can also make blood more sticky and likely to clot, which can lead to a blockage in an artery and a heart attack.

HRT and Heart Disease

It used to be thought that taking HRT containing estrogen might help lower your risk of heart disease, but large studies of more than 20,000 women clearly show this is not the case. In fact, research now shows that HRT slightly increases your risk of heart disease and stroke.

Research File

Several studies over the past few years show that including soy in your diet may help protect against heart disease by lowering cholesterol levels, which is an important breakthrough in medicine for post-menopausal women who are no longer protected by estrogen.

It was discovered almost by accident in the late 1960s that soy protein lowers cholesterol levels. Researchers who were looking at whether soy could be a palatable alternative protein to meat discovered a marked reduction in cholesterol levels in people who consumed a lot of soy.

Almost a decade later, Dr Sitori at the University of Milan discovered that soy protein lowered cholesterol levels by an average of 14% within two weeks and 21% within three weeks.

In 1999, Dr Kenneth Carrol analysed the results of 40 published studies on the effects of soy on cholesterol. He found that 34 of the studies showed a drop in levels of bad (LDL) cholesterol by 15% or more.

The Italians are so convinced about the value of soy in lowering cholesterol that it is now provided free of charge by the Italian National Health Service to people with high cholesterol.

Another study in the US by Professor Kenneth Setchell reported at the Third International Symposium on The Role of Soy in Preventing and Treating Chronic Disease in Washington DC confirmed that it is possible to raise HDL, while lowering LDL. The 12-week study on 43 post-menopausal women consuming a soy-rich diet containing 60-70mg of total isoflavones each day highlighted the antioxidant effects of soy.

On 20 October 1999, the US Food and Drug Administration (FDA) approved a health claim for soy protein and its role in reducing the risk of coronary heart disease. This same endorsement was eventually granted by the UK authorities. This means it can be stated on the label of food products containing at least 6.25mg of soy protein per serving that the product may reduce the risk of heart disease when consumed in conjunction with a low-fat, low-cholesterol diet.

A multi-center study published in December 2005 suggests that soy-enriched foods may help protect women from heart disease after menopause by reducing inflammation. It is thought that before menopause, estrogen protects women from heart disease by lowering the amount of such inflammatory markers in the blood. Some 117 European women were given either isoflavone-enriched or normal cereal bars. The results of the study suggest that soy protects some women more than others, depending on their genetic make-up.

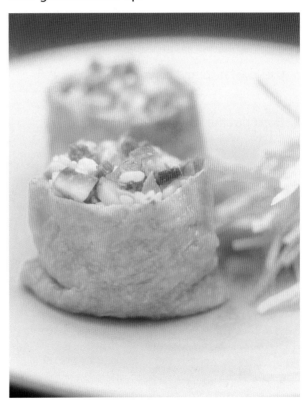

5 'Hearty' Things to Do Today

1. Leave your car at home and walk to the supermarket or work

2. Go for a 20-minute walk at lunch time

3. Listen to some music and get dancing

4. Use low-fat spread on your toast

5. Don't put the salt shaker on the table

Did You Know?

According to research in 1990 at the University of California, diet can be as effective in combating atherosclerosis as drugs or surgery. In the study, a group of people with severely blocked arteries went on a very low-fat vegetarian diet and exercise and meditation program, at the end of which their arteries were clear of plaque.

Research suggests that isoflavones can reduce the risk of coronary heart disease. A meta-analysis of the effects of soy protein containing isoflavones on blood lipids showed beneficial reductions in serum total cholesterol, LDL-cholesterol and triglycerides, with increased beneficial HDL-cholesterol.

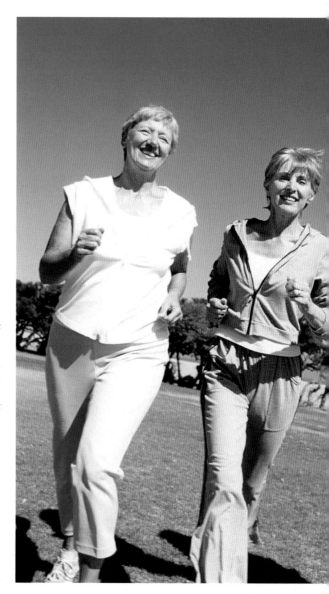

Jean's story

Jean Cunningham is a retired civil servant from Glasgow. Apart from other symptoms, she had a history of high blood pressure and an elevated cholesterol level.

I approached the NHAS for help with my headaches and fatigue, which had become worse since taking HRT. I changed my diet as instructed, including foods that contained naturally occurring estrogen, phytoestrogen-rich supplements, and began taking regular exercise and relaxation. After only a few weeks, I had so much more energy and my friends commented on how clear my skin looked. I'd been treated for high blood pressure and both my consultant and my doctor were amazed to discover that, since embarking on the NHAS program, my blood pressure had dropped into the normal range and my cholesterol level had reduced from 5.9 to 5.4.

133

"There is no need to mourn the loss of your reproductive years.
Once a woman has overcome the physical symptoms of menopause,
she can embrace the wonders that lie ahead for her.
This can be such a positive time."

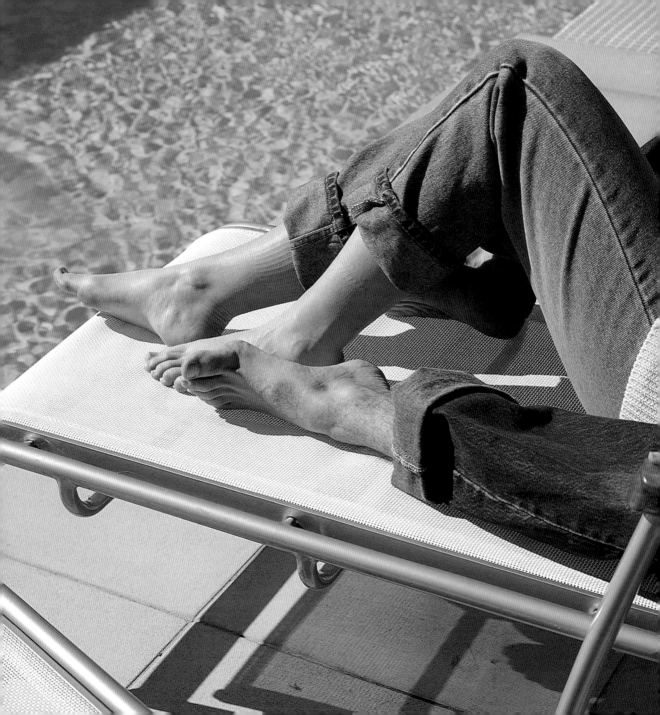

rev up your sex life

Your partner is eager, but sex is the last thing on your mind. Before you start thinking this is something peculiar to you, rest assured you are not alone. Many women find that their desire for sex starts to wane as they go into menopause. According to the American Medical Association a recent study revealed that 45% or 40 million women in the USA felt that their sex drive had reduced since menopause.

Tiredness, lack of energy and mood swings can put a dampener on the most solid relationship. At the same time, falling levels of estrogen can result in the lining of your vagina becoming dry and uncomfortable. When the vaginal tissues dry out, penetration can become painful and, in extreme cases, can result in tearing and bleeding. If you are also suffering from night sweats, it's not surprising that you don't feel much like having sex.

Many women suffer in silence, thinking this is an inevitable part of growing older. But the good news is it doesn't have to be this way. There are plenty of things you can do to naturally repair the vaginal lining, encourage the cells to produce mucus again and get your libido back.

Start by answering Yes or No to the following questions:

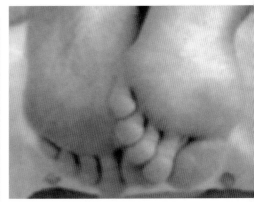

	Yes	No
Have you lost your sex drive?	☐	☐
Do you have sex less often than you used to?	☐	☐
Do you find sex painful?	☐	☐
Does your vagina feel dry?	☐	☐
Have you stopped looking forward to sex?	☐	☐
Have you stopped communicating with your lover on an intimate level?	☐	☐
Are you too tired for sex?	☐	☐
Has your enjoyment of sex diminished?	☐	☐
Do you make excuses in order to avoid sex?	☐	☐

If you answered Yes to more than two of these questions, try the following Action Plan to give your sex life a boost. Remember to enter your score on the Natural Menopause Plan on page 322.

Gladys' Story

Gladys Sellars had been experiencing menopausal symptoms for over two years. She suffered with hot flashes and night sweats, which would overtake her whole body to such an extent that she thought she was going mad. Her vagina was so dry that she couldn't bear to be touched.

I developed very bad headaches, aches and pains, depression, irritability and moodiness. I was afraid to go out by myself because I was so nervous. I had an incredibly dry vagina and sex had become so painful that I didn't want to be touched. I saw Maryon Stewart talking on TV and realised that I wasn't going mad and that all the symptoms I had were due to menopause. I used to take it all out on my husband – I know that was wrong – but I couldn't help it. I was lucky he was so supportive and encouraged me to see Maryon.

I went to see Maryon, answered her questions and explained my symptoms, which she confirmed were associated with menopause. She wrote a program for me that involved making specific dietary changes, including naturally-occurring estrogen in my diet, plus scientifically based supplements like Gynovite, Promensil and Omega-7. I also started using Phyto Soya Gel to

help with my dry vagina and started daily exercise and formal relaxation.

I followed the recommendations and, by the time I went back to Maryon one month later, I was feeling significantly different. The hot flashes and night sweats had become mild. Maryon reviewed my progress, gave me a pat on the back and sent me off to continue the program for another month. By the next visit, the fatigue, irritability, anxiety, nervous tension and loss of confidence had completely gone. I was hardly experiencing any symptoms at all, except for a few hot flashes and some mild aches and pains. Maryon reviewed my program again and, within four months of starting her program, I was completely symptom-free. I had also lost 3kg without dieting.

I began driving a car again and I felt so much better. I wasn't nervous any more and I was no longer afraid to go shopping by myself. I was able to be a good mother again, rather than shut off in my own world, and got back to being a good wife as I no longer had a dry vagina and we were once again able to enjoy our personal life. Everyone has noticed the difference in how I look and feel. I'm so glad that I managed to get through my menopause naturally, without resorting to HRT.

Action Plan

Assess Your Diet

Our research shows it is important to correct nutritional deficiencies and consume a nutrient-dense, isoflavone-rich diet to help put yourself on a more even keel emotionally.

Supplement it

There are several specific supplements that have been shown in clinical trials to help boost libido and repair dry vaginal tissue. These include Omega-7 (Sea Buckthorn Oil) and Phyto Soya Gel.

Get in Touch

Treat each other to a sensual massage. Turn on some music, dim the lights and start gently touching each other. Essential oils, such as jasmine, rose, ylang ylang, clary sage or sandalwood, may heighten your experience.

Talk to Each Other

Expecting your partner to understand what is going on, without you explaining, is an easy trap to fall into and can quickly put a distance between you. Try to spend some time together to explain what you are going through. Ask for his support.

Say it with Flowers

If your relationship is less than healthy, a dose of Bach Flower Remedies may help bring back that loving feeling. Wild Rose remedy is believed to renew interest in life and boost vitality, while Olive is thought to have revitalizing properties. Larch is the one to go for if you have lost confidence in your ability to make love.

Experiment

If penetration is really painful, explore other avenues of giving each other pleasure. Go back to your courting days and indulge in plenty of foreplay. There is no need to shy away from using a lubricant. The important thing is that you continue to communicate physically and emotionally.

"Before starting the NHAS program, my vagina used to bleed and it felt like a hot ball of fire. I now take Omega-7 capsules and insert Phyto Soya Gel twice a week. Amazingly, my vaginal tissues feel completely different."
Lynn Carr

Diane's Story

Diane, 50, had been suffering with her symptoms for seven years before she approached the NHAS.

I was still working full-time in the education department of our local government office. The first menopausal symptom I experienced was that I was finding it harder and harder to concentrate. This led to a lack of self-confidence, which affected my performance at work and my home life.

I had to take time off and get others to stand in for me, since jobs that should have taken me five minutes were taking hours. I had always loved my career, but for the first time in my life, I was thinking of giving it up.

I started to feel constantly ill, with migraine headaches and repeated hot flashes. I felt like I had hit rock-bottom emotionally and everything seemed to be a chore. I felt old, haggard and undesirable and seemed to have aged inside and out almost overnight. To say my self-esteem was at an all-time low would be an understatement!

My husband had always been very supportive, but my irrational behavior and my loss of libido were putting quite a strain on our relationship. I knew my behavior was unacceptable, so I went to see my doctor and was prescribed antidepressants. They didn't work and made me feel that I was not only experiencing menopausal symptoms, but also that I was mentally ill. Still feeling low, I saw another doctor and was prescribed HRT.

For six months, I felt on top of the world. Most of my symptoms disappeared, although my libido didn't fully recover. Then the migraines returned with a vengeance. Once again, I couldn't sleep and was feeling sick and suffering with dairrhea. My legs felt like lead. I had no energy at all and I had terrible sugar cravings. I actually took myself off HRT and contacted the NHAS for help.

I made specific dietary changes, began taking the recommended nutritional supplements and exercised regularly. Within two weeks, the hot flashes had stopped. My migraine headaches lifted and, within a short space of time, my whole attitude to life became more positive. From lying in bed feeling depressed, I noticed that, come morning, I wanted to jump out of bed and get on with the day, just like I had when I was younger. Once again, I had lots of energy, my moods were much more constant and I no longer felt irrational. Thankfully, my libido returned and I resumed a normal, loving relationship with my husband. I felt more confident and enjoyed laughing again. It felt like I had been released from a prison!

It's been eight years now and I still feel absolutely brilliant. I'm delighted with the progress I've made. My husband was very relieved too, as he felt so helpless at the time. Within six months, I was a totally different person and I've never looked back. I need far less sleep now. I took a university degree and learned to play the piano. I feel tremendous, like a new woman. Best of all, I look like one too!

Survey Results

NHAS Menopause Relationship Survey
Sponsored by Arkopharma

In April 2004, we analysed the results of the Menopause Relationship Survey, which had been on our website for a few months. To appreciate the difficulty of getting a real understanding of the extent of the problem, it is worth mentioning that although 6,991 women visited the website and opened the survey, only 1,160 women were willing to share their problems and complete the questionnaire. After reviewing the completed responses, 673 women were identified as being menopausal. Of these, 353 hadn't had a period within the last six months, nor were they taking HRT.

The results clearly showed that menopause often has a major effect on personal relationships. From the sample of 673 women who completed the survey, we discovered:

Strain on Relationship

66% cent of women said that menopause put a strain on their relationship, with 37% saying their relationship was moderately to severely affected.

Loss of Libido

59% of women experienced a loss of libido at the time of menopause. 29% experienced this to a moderate to severe degree. Of the 353 HRT users, 30% saw no benefit with respect to their loss of libido and 4% said it was made worse on HRT.

Orgasm

50% of women had difficulty achieving orgasm.

Dry Vagina

55% of women had a dry vagina. 42% of women who took HRT said it did not help 'more than slightly' with vaginal dryness.

Painful Intercourse

36% of women suffered from painful intercourse and 47% admitted a lack of sexual sensations.

The findings clearly showed that menopausal women have problems with libido and sex. Our experience at the NHAS suggests these problems are probably related to underlying nutritional deficiencies that prevent the brain chemistry from working properly. This has a domino effect with sex hormone function.

HRT users had fewer problems, but still experienced painful intercourse. Since HRT is no longer regarded as a long-term option, it is important for women to know that they can overcome their symptoms naturally by following a program such as our Natural Menopause Plan.

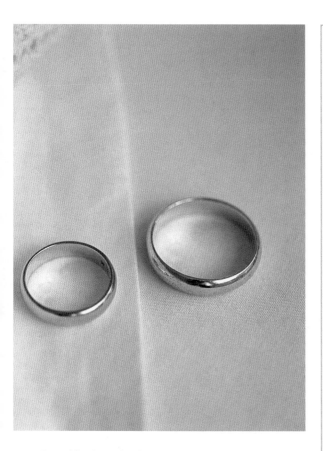

"My libido, which was non-existent, has completely returned and my husband has made it known that he is delighted to have his wife back."
Rosanna Haslam

"I'm back at university training as a speech therapist doing things that were beyond my dreams... Now I'm heading to a very bright future."

Mairin Gallagher

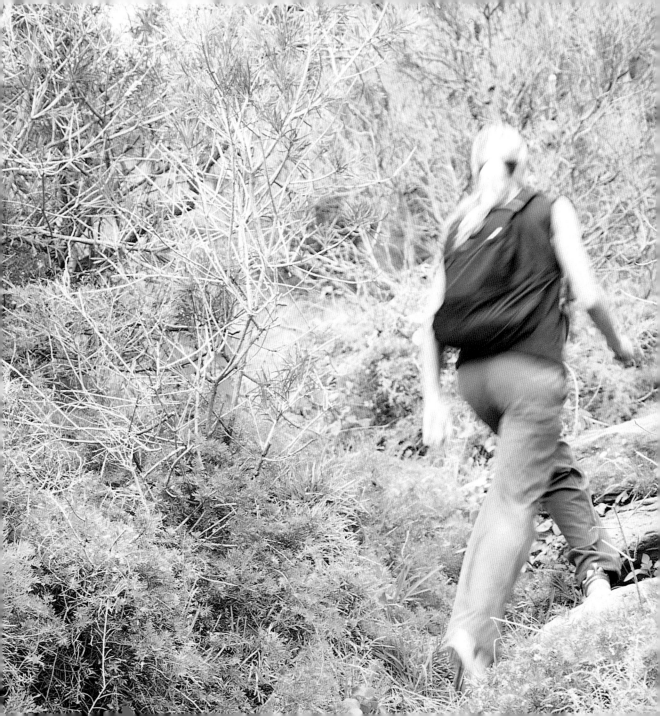

regain your zest for life

Imagine if a new drug came on the market offering increased mental alertness, more energy and vitality, the ability to perform daily tasks without getting breathless or tired, more flexibility, faster reaction times, increased immunity and stronger bones. The shops would be inundated!

Well, the good news is, this 'drug' already exists. It's called 'exercise' and it can be yours for little or no cost. Perhaps the only drawback is that, unlike a magic pill, you have to put in some time and effort to achieve the benefits, but this is a small price to pay for such huge rewards.

Before you say you're too old to start an exercise regime, remember that it's even more important to be positive about exercise now than when you were younger. Anything that gets you moving will help improve your energy levels, symptoms of depression, anxiety and insomnia, as well as boost your confidence, self-esteem and wellbeing.

Aerobic exercise - anything that makes you feel hot and slightly out of breath - helps protect against heart disease. Weight-bearing exercise - supporting your own body weight, such as Pilates or yoga, or using weights for extra resistance - helps strengthen your bones and protects against osteoporosis (see p122 for specific exercises).

Exercise is very important at this time of your life as your metabolism (the rate at which your body burns calories) tends to slow down as you get older. When you were young, you could probably eat what you liked without gaining much weight, but now you only have to look at a doughnut to pile on the kilos, especially around the middle.

Exercise helps in several ways. Firstly, you burn calories while you're doing it, and it can also increase your metabolic rate for up to 24 hours afterwards. Secondly, regular exercise, particularly strength or resistance training, builds muscle. The greater your muscle mass, the higher your metabolic rate and the more calories you burn.

If you really dislike exercise, you're probably already groaning, but I promise you will reap enormous benefits from getting up and moving. Many women who started exercise for the first time as part of the NHAS program have come to absolutely love it. If you need further encouragement, remember that exercise also improves your circulation, so your skin will look better, making you feel more radiant and youthful.

If the thought of exercising makes you want to skip to the next chapter, don't worry, you're not expected to run a marathon (unless you want to, of course). You're only competing with yourself. The aim is to improve your level of fitness gradually over a period of months.

1 Firstly, if you haven't exercised for a long time, check with your doctor before starting any exercise program. This also applies if you suffer from heart disease, have high blood pressure, joint problems, back problems, are very overweight, have a serious illness or are convalescing.

2 Before performing any exercises in your home or in your garden, check that the location is safe and that the surfaces are not wet or slippery.

3 Make sure you are warm enough, with layered, loose clothing that can be discarded as you heat up.

4 Ensure that the support and equipment you use is strong enough to take your weight.

5 Don't exercise for at least an hour after meals, and drink plenty of water to avoid becoming dehydrated.

How Fit Are You?

To assess your current level of fitness, answer Yes or No to the following questions:

	Yes	No
Do you exercise?	☐	☐
Are you currently doing some exercise occasionally?	☐	☐
Do you exercise more than three times a week for more than 30 minutes at a time?	☐	☐
Does it take a lot of exercise before you feel breathless?	☐	☐
Can you run up and down stairs without panting?	☐	☐

If you answered No to more than two of these questions, you need to get started on our Natural Menopause Plan now. Remember to enter your score on the Natural Menopause Plan on page 322.

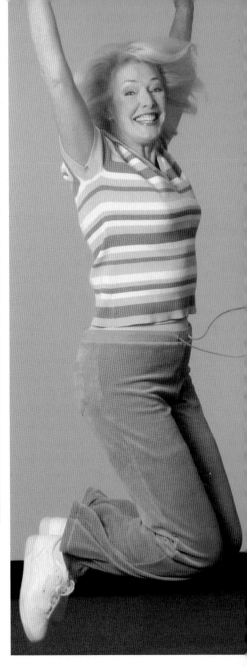

Action Plan

The first rule of exercise is to choose something you enjoy. If you already like walking on a treadmill or along a country lane, this is a great place to start. If you don't like any exercise, think back to activities you enjoyed when you were younger. Maybe you were a whiz at tennis, swimming, dancing or roller skating. There are more and more activities available today for people of all ages, so you should be able to find something that suits you.

You may prefer to exercise with a friend or in a group. This might mean joining an exercise or dance class, going for a jog with a friend, selecting a good home exercise DVD or simply dancing or singing to your favorite music. Whatever it takes and whatever you fancy, you have already jumped the most difficult hurdle - you've started.

Once you start, it's a good idea to vary the type of exercise you do on different days of the week to target different parts of your body and help stave off boredom. Good options include running, power walking, cycling, swimming, cardiovascular machines at the gym, tennis, squash, badminton, dancing, rope-skipping or an aerobics-based exercise class.

Alternatively, you can just stretch and dance to your favorite music. I tune in to Planet Rock on my digital radio and do a workout before the day begins and I swear I feel 20 years younger as a result. If you haven't got an established exercise routine, I recommend you give it a try.

How Long and How Often?

The second rule of exercise is to start slowly, otherwise you risk discomfort or injury, especially if you're not used to exercise. 'A little and often' should be the rule. The old adage of 'no pain, no gain' is also outdated. Exercise does not have to be hell to be healthy.

You should feel invigorated at the end of your activity, but not exhausted. It is important to listen to your body at all times. Sometimes you will have plenty of energy and feel you can tackle anything, sometimes you won't. The secret is not to push yourself too hard, just do as much as you feel comfortable with.

The general consensus is that women entering menopause and beyond should aim to exercise regularly four or five times a week for 30 to 60 minutes (provided they don't suffer from cardiovascular disease) and that they should build up to this gradually over a period of at least three months.

Keep the benefits of exercise uppermost in your mind until you have established a regular routine. When you reach your goal of four or five exercise sessions a week, try to maintain it. There's no need to do more - too much exercise can be bad for you, putting a strain on your joints and bones.

After each workout, tap into how you are feeling. Exercise encourages your body to release endorphins, the body's own feel-good hormones that make you feel elated, full of energy and proud of yourself. Hold on to that feeling and, next time you start talking yourself out of your daily exercise, remind yourself of how good it makes you feel.

Watch Points

1 Remember to warm up and cool down after exercising.

2 Warm up slowly for the first few minutes.

3 Continue exercising until you reach the point of breathlessness - this is the signal to start cooling down.

4 Take a few moments to cool down gradually, rather than stopping suddenly.

5 Ways to Sneak Exercise into Your Day

1. Walk around while talking to friends on the phone or during the ad breaks on TV.

2. Use the stairs, not the elevator.

3. Put down the TV remote control and get up off the sofa to change channels.

4. Leave your car behind and walk or run to collect the newspapers.

5. Put some real effort into housework.

Within 12 weeks of starting an exercise regime, you will feel more energetic, cope more effectively with stress, sleep better, fight off infections more successfully and generally feel a whole lot better.

Warm-up Moves

Whatever type of exercise you choose, you must warm up before you start. This helps get you in the mood and also encourages blood flow to your muscles, providing oxygen to fuel your activities. Walking, gentle jogging, marching on the spot, cycling or any activity that uses your large muscle groups are good warm-up moves.

You need to move your joints through their full range of movement to loosen them up and to gently stretch the muscles you are about to use. Try to hold your stretches for six to eight seconds, and avoid bouncing if you can.

Exercise Increases

- high density lipoproteins (HDLs), the good cholesterol

- oxygen transport

- aerobic capacity

- circulation

- bone mass and density

- reaction time and coordination

- energy levels

- overall wellbeing

Exercise Decreases

- low density lipoproteins (LDLs), the bad cholesterol

- risk of heart disease

- blood pressure

- body fat

- anxiety, stress and depression

- risk of diabetes

Cool-Down Moves

Exercise increases your heart rate, making you breathe faster and deeper, which is good for heart health. But in the same way as you use gears to gradually slow down a car, it is much better to come out of exercise gradually, rather than stopping suddenly.

Gently stretch the muscles that you have been using, to keep them flexible. Try to build in some relaxation time at the end of your session to reward yourself for your efforts and to give you time to release tension.

Research File

A recent study showed that pre-menopausal women with an average age of 41 who trained for nine weeks improved their oxygen intake by 12%, while post-menopausal women improved their oxygen intake by 19%.

In another study, women who undertook a 12-week walking and jogging program felt better, enjoyed social functions more, participated in more activities and were not as tired at the end of the day. One researcher, Spiriduso, concluded that, "Exercise seems to be one way for people to achieve maximal plasticity in aging, approximating full vigour and consistency of performance."

Exercise has been shown to improve symptoms of depression and anxiety more effectively than psychotherapy. In a comparative study, after a 12-week aerobic program, the women who exercised had fewer symptoms of depression and anxiety than women who had psychotherapy. At the follow-up session one year later, this was still the case.

Exercise may even offset aging of the central nervous system. People who exercise regularly are consistently more alert and have faster reaction times. It has also been shown that the fitter people are, the more competent they are likely to be.

According to a new study published in the Journal of Advanced Nursing, regular exercise can reduce severe menopausal symptoms and improve quality of life. Researchers from the University of Granada in Spain found that the number of women suffering severe symptoms dropped nearly 25% after they began a 12-month, supervised exercise program consisting of cardio respiratory, stretching, muscle-strengthening and relaxation exercises, while symptoms worsened among women who didn't exercise.

Active women tend to suffer less from menopausal symptoms. Sustained, regular aerobic exercise, such as swimming, walking, cycling and running, tend to work best.

Q Why does exercise makes me sweat, or is it a hot flash?

A If you're not used to exercise, you may start to sweat. It's not just another hot flash, but a sign that your body is using up energy and needs to get rid of the excess heat it is producing. Sweating does not mean you are unfit, but the reverse - the fitter you become, the more efficient your body becomes at removing excess sweat.

Q Should I worry if I huff and puff?

A You may start to huff and puff if you're working hard, but as long as you can still carry on a conversation and are not in any distress, this should be nothing to worry about. It just means you're working!

"I thought I'd lost my sex drive…
Now I have it all back and I'm feeling wonderful!"

Sharyn McLaughlin

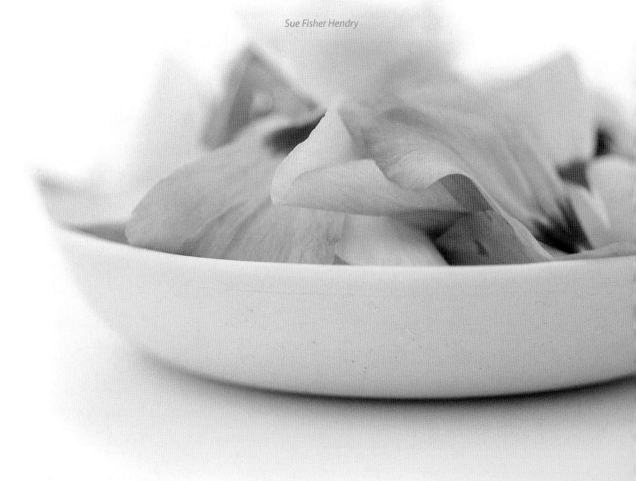

Trying to find a quick fix to the emotional side of menopause is as unnatural as trying to pretend puberty doesn't happen!

Sue Fisher Hendry

think positive

At the time of menopause, our attitudes and emotions play a big part in how we feel. As Sue Fisher Hendry points out in our DVD, it's not just our own attitudes, but also those of society that influence us as we age. As we prepare for midlife, we enter brand new territory. In addition to the physical changes occurring in our bodies, many of us find that the onset of perimenopause, menopause and the aging process all challenge our attitudes and emotions.

You may, for example, start to think you're invisible. You no longer turn heads as you walk down the street and builders seem strangely silent at the top of their ladders - gone are the wolf-whistle days. As a result, you may start to feel unattractive, a feeling not helped by the attitude of many men that you are now just a 'woman of a certain age'.

At the end of the day, it's more about how you feel about yourself and whether your 'lamp' is switched on as to how attractive you appear. If you feel well, healthy and are in good shape it will be reflected in your skin, hair and nails, there will be a spring in your step and that old sparkle in your eyes will be alive and well. But if you let yourself go physically as well as mentally, then menopause can feel like the beginning of the end, instead of an entirely new beginning. If you have lost your grip along the way, it is possible to reframe your attitudes and get back to being your old self or even better.

Our attitudes are affected in a number of ways as we enter midlife. They can be broken down into the messages and attitudes that come from within us as individuals, and the messages and attitudes that come from the world around us.

Attitudes can be both positive and negative. Some women are delighted to be done with having periods and are happy to grow older gracefully. Other women are horrified by the process, mourning the loss of their reproductive years and worrying that 'it's all downhill from here'.

Many women are affected by the advertising and media coverage they see on a daily basis, which mostly sends the message that young and beautiful women are much more valuable in our society than older, wiser women.

In 1998, we conducted a survey at the NHAS into women's attitudes at the time of menopause. Although 80% of women surveyed were delighted their periods had stopped, 40% were anxious and afraid of their physical appearance, 37% felt that menopause signalled the start of old age, and a worrying 17% thought their partner would prefer a younger woman!

These results make depressing reading, yet most of them can be termed as 'crooked' thinking because, once the physical symptoms of menopause have been overcome and fatigue is no longer an issue,

the midlife years can be an enormously positive phase in your life. They should be seen not so much as the death of the reproductive years, but as the beginning or rebirth of a whole new you. Ideally, you need to spend less time hanging around the fountain of youth and more time bathing in the waters of wisdom!

The first step to changing the way you think is to learn to love yourself for what you are and to accept the stage of life you are in. The secret is to embrace midlife, not run away from it.

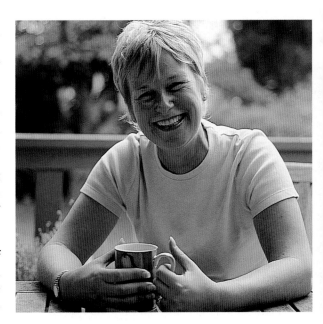

How Do You See Yourself?

To find out where you stand in the self-worth stakes, answer Yes or No (as honestly as you can!)

	Yes	No
Do you feel unattractive?	☐	☐
Do you think life as you once knew it is over?	☐	☐
Do you see yourself as old?	☐	☐
Do you see menopause as the beginning of the end?	☐	☐
Do you think your partner (if you have one) no longer finds you attractive?	☐	☐
Do you think your partner would prefer to be with a younger woman?	☐	☐
Do you think you are now too old to find a partner? (if appropriate)	☐	☐
Do you tend to concentrate on your bad points, rather than your good points?	☐	☐

	Yes	No
Do you tend to dwell on your failures, rather than your achievements?	☐	☐
Are you unhappy with what you have achieved in life?	☐	☐
Do you sometimes doubt your ability to succeed?	☐	☐
Do you see life as all downhill from now on?	☐	☐
Do you wish you were young again?	☐	☐
Do you think you were more attractive when you were younger?	☐	☐
Do you think you are too old for good sex?	☐	☐
Do you dread menopause?	☐	☐
Do you dread having more free time?	☐	☐

If you answer Yes to more than three questions, it's time to change your attitudes and start feeling good about yourself again, so get going on our Natural Menopause Plan. Make a note of your score on page 322. It will be useful to compare it with your 'after' score, which you will complete in three month's time.

Action Plan

Create Some 'Me' Time

The first key to an emotionally healthy and rewarding midlife is to examine the attitudes that affect you. You need to spend some time working out what your priorities and values are at this time of life. They will probably be very different from what they were 10 years ago. It's important you find time to get to know yourself again, as well as time to laugh and share friendships. It is vital that you never lose your precious sense of humor.

It is also vital to achieve a relaxed 'head space'. Both the physical and emotional symptoms of menopause are made significantly worse by stress, so relaxation and meditation techniques are a must. You should find an hour each day to exercise, relax or meditate.

How to be Future Positive

Being optimistic about the future is more likely to bring results than thinking about how good things were. There is lots of evidence to show that those who see life as a 'glass half-full', rather than a 'glass half-empty', stand a much better chance of feeling content and fulfilled as they go into midlife. So if your thoughts are veering towards the negative, indulge in some positive thinking when you wake up and before you go to sleep at night. Form a vivid picture of your happy, attractive self going through the rest of life being incredibly positive and start looking at things through these positive eyes. You'll feel so much better about life!

Spend time imagining yourself in great physical and mental shape, looking and feeling great with good things happening to you. Maybe now that the children have left home, you are starting to recreate the romance of those first heady days you spent with your partner, or you're enjoying the company of new friends or even starting a new relationship. Perhaps your daydreams will center on success in your work or even going back to work or starting a new hobby or fulfilling a lifetime ambition or dream.

Whatever you decide to focus on, make the images in your mind so realistic that you actually start to feel you are experiencing the situation. It may take some practice, but once you get the hang of it, it will become like watching a movie. Remember that unless you feel positive about yourself, you don't stand much of a chance of people reacting in a positive way towards you.

Pat Yourself on the Back

It also helps to keep a note of your daily achievements, however small. It is all too easy to move on to the next thing, or even the next day, without acknowledging what you have accomplished. Again, we tend to fixate on the negative, our mistakes and things that perhaps we later regret. Making time to review your successes helps you build self-confidence. Get yourself a notebook and write in it on a daily basis as you would a diary. Read back over it each week and congratulate yourself on how well you are doing.

Make Yourself Proud

It's all too easy to go from one day to the next without considering the needs of others. The rewards that come from helping make other people's lives more pleasant are priceless. Team up with a friend who is also going through menopause and you can give each other help and encouragement. You'll be surprised how much of a buzz it will give you. It can also help to know that you're not alone and that other women are going through menopause too and feel just like you.

Live Your Dream

You won't realize your dreams without making an effort. Some people say there's no point in dreaming because fate takes charge of your destiny! Evidence shows you can get what you wish for by applying specific techniques. Positive thinking and visualization can go a long way to getting you where you would like to be and helping you change your attitudes, especially when it comes to turning negatives into positives.

Take five or ten minutes out each day to visualize yourself the way you would like to be. Experts believe the best time for this is first thing in the morning and last thing at night, so start and finish your day visualizing yourself just the way you would like to be - happy, fulfilled, looking forward to good things in the future or whatever takes your fancy. Visualization is an acquired skill, so if it doesn't immediately happen in technicolour

and your mind keeps wandering, stick with it, eventually you will get it. You have nothing to lose and it's a positive way to begin and end each day.

As well as visualizing, make a collage of your dream with clippings from magazines to help focus on your goals. This is a fun activity that allows you to create your life the way you want it and design your dreams. It beats sitting around waiting for things to happen to you or just accepting what comes your way. We hold collage workshops on the website at www.askmaryonstewart.com so look out for them. In the meantime, remember that there is a great deal of good living to be enjoyed in this new and exciting phase of your life, but you have to recognize that you are the architect of your life, not a victim of circumstances!

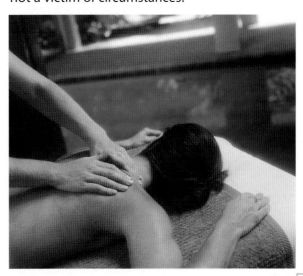

"People could hardly believe I was the same person. I can't describe how much difference the program has made to my life!"

Zoe Howes

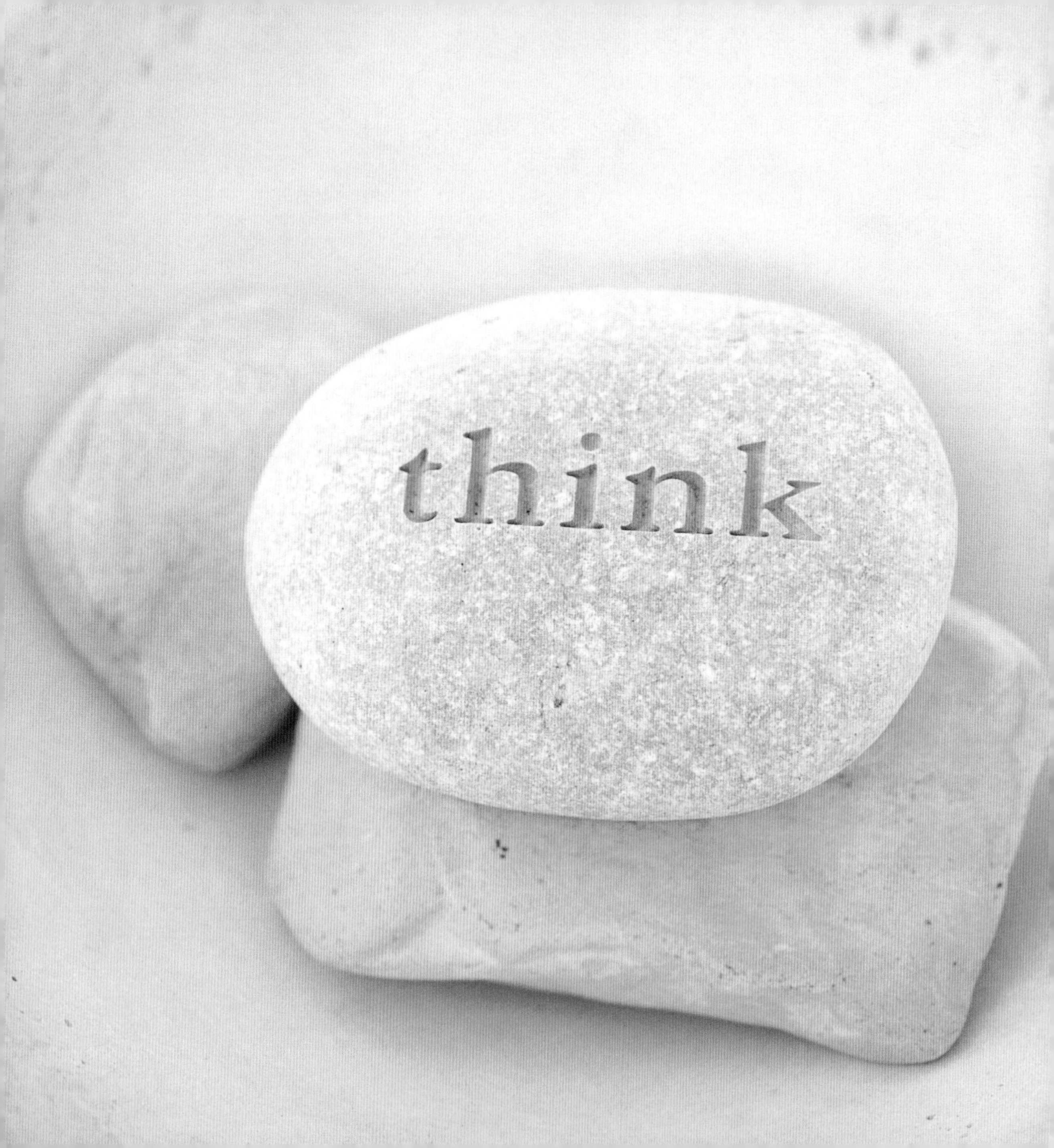
think

boost your brain power

Do you lose your train of thought mid-sentence, forget where you left your keys or what you went upstairs for? You may have 'senior moments', but you're not losing your marbles. We all start to forget things as we age, say the experts. When asked to memorize a list of 75 words read out five times, the average 18-year-old scores 54, a 45-year-old scores 47 and a 65-year-old scores just 37.

And the reason? No-one knows for sure, but it's thought most memory problems at this time of life are due to poor concentration, lack of motivation, tiredness, anxiety or stress, rather than loss of brain cells. Feeling fuzzy-headed is also thought to be related to the hormonal ups and downs associated with menopause. Some parts of the brain particularly involved with verbal memory are rich in estrogen receptors, so there could be a genuine physiological link between hormonal status and brain function. This is confirmed by research undertaken by Dr Sandra File at Guy's Hospital in London.

As we grow older, our circulation slows down, thus less oxygen reaches our brain cells, so it's no surprise we aren't as sharp. Many of us don't stretch our brains as much as we could. Like muscles, our brain needs to be used to function at optimum levels. The good news is forgetfulness doesn't have to be an inevitable part of getting older. Following a nutrient-dense and phytoestrogen-rich diet, leading an active lifestyle and keeping your brain well exercised will help keep you sharp.

To assess just how on-the-ball you are, start boosting your mental powers by answering Yes or No to the following questions:

	Yes	No
Do you ever forget what you went upstairs for?	☐	☐
Can you remember telephone numbers?	☐	☐
Do you find it hard to concentrate?	☐	☐
Do you find you forget a person's name the moment after you've been introduced?	☐	☐
Are you prone to absent-minded acts, such as putting milk in the cupboard?	☐	☐
Have you ever missed an appointment because you forgot it?	☐	☐
Do you have to write arrangements down the minute you make them for fear of forgetting them?	☐	☐
Have you ever forgotten the name of someone you know well?	☐	☐
Do you frequently lose your car keys?	☐	☐
Have you ever forgotten what you were saying mid-sentence?	☐	☐
Have you ever gone to mention something important to someone, but gone completely bank?	☐	☐
Have you ever put something in the oven and forgotten to take it out?	☐	☐
Have you ever said you would do something for someone, but completely forgotten to do it?	☐	☐

If you answered 'Yes' to more than three questions, it's time to try some memory-boosting foods and supplements, as well as doing some mental exercises. Don't forget to enter your score on page 322.

Action Plan

• The brain is dependent on glucose, essential fats and phospholipids for good health. Several B vitamins are also essential for normal memory and mental performance. Zinc and magnesium are necessary for neuro-transmitter metabolism. So it follows that including certain nutrients in your diet can help boost your concentration, attention span, as well as short-term and long-term memory. Current research also suggests that brain-boosting supplements can help improve your memory skills.

• Ginkgo Biloba, a herbal extract made from the leaves of the Chinese maidenhair tree, has gained recognition over the past 30 years as a brain tonic that helps restore vascular function and memory.

• More than 300 medical studies have been published, most indicating the benefits of taking daily supplements. Ginkgo improves circulation, which in turn increases blood flow, carrying more nutrients and oxygen to the brain. This helps restore short-term and long-term memory, helping you think more clearly and concentrate better.

• Foods rich in the antioxidant Vitamins A, C and E help mop up free radicals, the rogue molecules that can cause excessive cell damage in the body, including the brain. Good sources include richly coloured vegetables, such as bananas, red peppers, spinach and oranges.

• Oily fish is rich in omega-3 fatty acids, as well as folic acid, all of which are vital for the smooth functioning of the brain and nervous system. Good sources include sardines, salmon, herring, pilchards and mackerel.

• In the past few years, research has confirmed that eating soy improves memory not just in the younger generation, but also in menopausal women. The estrogen-like effects of isoflavones have led to speculation that soy may also help maintain cognitive function in older women and reduce the risk of Alzheimer's disease.

• A healthy diet, regular exercise, not smoking and watching what you drink will help keep your brain sharp and reduce your risk of dementia.

A healthy diet, regular exercise, not smoking and watching what you drink will help keep your brain sharp and reduce your risk of dementia.

Many studies show that stimulation is the key to good memory and that people who take part in lots of different types of activity have better powers of recall. The more active your brain is, the better your memory is likely to be, and the more different ways you use your mind, the easier you'll find it to remember things. It's all to do with being active, rather than passive: whether you actively concentrate and focus on things or whether you just let them wash over you. Try the following exercises to sharpen your mental faculties:

- Do a mental exercise every day – a crossword, Sudoko, word search or quiz. If you don't know the answer, look it up, then try to remember it the next day.

- When doing your finances, put away the calculator and use your brain instead.

- Take up new activities – gardening, knitting or anything active involving your hand-eye or foot-eye coordination.

- Make shopping lists, then memorize them before going to the shops.

- Engage in activities that stretch your brain, such as chess, bridge or anything that pushes you that little bit further.

- Work for as long as you can, keep up with your friends and join local social groups. Studies have shown that people who have plenty of friends, especially at work, do significantly better in memory and concentration tests than those who don't.

Did You Know?

Even if we fed information into our brain every second of our lives, it would not even be half-full when we die.

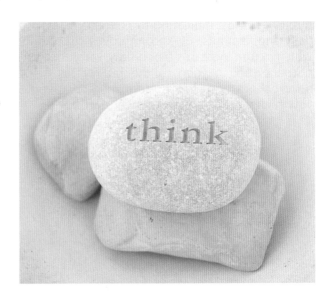

168

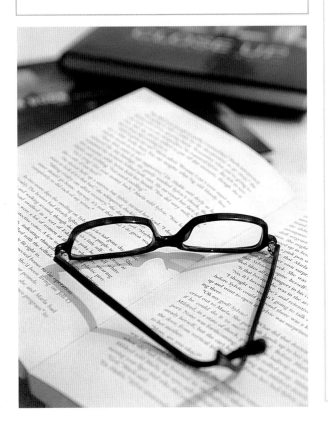

Nicola's Story

Nicola is a 46-year-old mother of two and part-time conference organizer.

I was only 44 when a blood test showed I was going through early menopause. I tried HRT, but within days started to feel panicky, depressed, out of control and - dare I say it - suicidal. I stopped taking HRT within the first week, but it took several months before I felt calm again. I went through hot and cold flashes, night sweats, headaches, abdominal bloating, constipation, general aches and pains, and depression.

At my first NHAS consultation, I was given advice about diet and supplements, which included eating phytoestrogen-rich foods and taking various supplements to boost my vitamin and mineral levels and help reduce my symptoms.

After just four months, I'm feeling so much better. I feel better mentally, my memory has returned and I feel more in control, as well as more positive about things. I don't feel so irritable and tired, and I'm sleeping much better. My flashes are not nearly so frequent and constipation has become a thing of the past.

I have also lost some weight without having to diet, which is a wonderful bonus. I am so pleased with myself and everyone says how much more rational I am now.

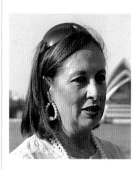

Sharyn's Story

Sharyn McLaughlin had a hysterectomy and started to take HRT. She had to be taken off it after only three months due to the adverse side-effects.

After having a hysterectomy, I went on HRT, but my breasts started to ache and I put on 6kg, so after six months I just stopped taking it one day. I started to feel hot and irritable and I found myself snapping at everyone, especially my staff. I wasn't usually moody, but I started to experience the most amazing mood swings and anxiety. My husband found me impossible to live with. I also couldn't remember a thing. Sometimes I would go places and couldn't remember why.

I started going to Maryon Stewart and thank goodness everything changed within a couple of months. I introduced soy to my diet and started taking Promensil, fish oils, calcium and magnesium. Everyone has noticed how much easier I am to be with now. I don't get so anxious and I don't forget things like I used to. I am much more content, I know where I'm going and I feel much more in control. I have learned to love myself and who I am.

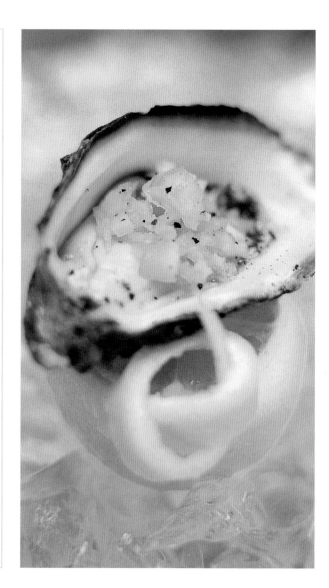

Research File

In a recent study of the elderly in the USA it was revealed that 5%-20% of elderly people, whether living at home or in institutions, may have a moderate to severe deficiency of Vitamin B12. An even higher percentage may suffer from deficiencies of other B vitamins. Depression can be associated with a lack of these important chemicals.

Vitamin E and other antioxidants may be important to help blood flow to the brain and central nervous system. A recent study showed patients with early signs of dementia improved after being given high doses of Vitamin E.

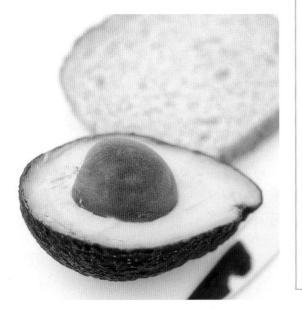

"People who take part in lots of different types of activity have better powers of recall."

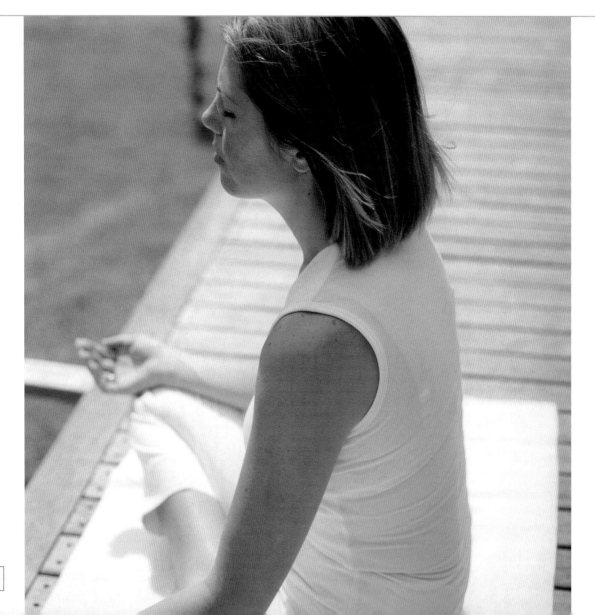

keep your cool

Life without challenges would be very dull, so in this sense a certain amount of stress can keep you on your toes. But too much stress is not a good thing, especially at this time of life, when you are being pulled mentally and physically in many directions. The pressure of balancing children, family, relationships, work and finances can take their toll. If you're not careful, stress can exacerbate symptoms such as flashes and sweats, leaving you feeling overwhelmed and under par.

The key to avoiding high stress levels is to have regular stress checks to ensure you keep a balance between good and bad stress. If the scales lean towards the bad, it's time to set in place a protective plan so your body is in the best possible state to stand up to any demands.

"I felt less stressed and much more like my normal self. I now look after two of my young grandchildren full-time and am amazed that I can cope. I never would have been able to before the program."
Mava Morrison

Take our stress test by answering Yes or No to the following questions:

	Yes	No		Yes	No
Are you tired all the time?	☐	☐	Do you have emotional problems?	☐	☐
Do you have trouble sleeping or wake up in the middle of the night?	☐	☐	Are your family relationships strained?	☐	☐
Do you crave sugary foods?	☐	☐	Are you forgetful?	☐	☐
Do you keep bursting into tears?	☐	☐	Is your digestive system upset?	☐	☐
Do you get frequent headaches?	☐	☐	Is your appetite reduced?	☐	☐
Do you find it hard to make up your mind?	☐	☐	Do you sometimes feel it's all too much?	☐	☐
Do you get butterflies in your stomach?	☐	☐	Do you find it difficult to communicate with people?	☐	☐
Do you feel anxious or on edge for no special reason?	☐	☐	Do you have too little time for yourself?	☐	☐

If you answered Yes to more than three of these questions, the chances are you're suffering from stress overload. If you scored more than six, you need to take some action to get back in the driver's seat. Remember to enter your score in your Natural Menopause Plan on page 322.

Action Plan

First you need to look at any obvious triggers and deal with them as best you can. Then you can get started on some simple stress management techniques to help reduce the pressure.

Keep things in perspective

Don't overreact to situations. Think realistically and talk through your problem with a friend. This can help you see it from an objective view point, rather than an irrational one, which can help lower stress levels.

Relax

Make time for relaxation, whether it be meditation or something as simple as soaking in a bath, listening to your favorite music, going for a walk or reading a book.

Eat well

Resist the temptation to reach for 'comfort' foods, such as chocolate, cakes, cookies, soft drinks and coffee. These interfere with your body's ability to absorb vitamins and minerals, often making you feel even worse. Eating foods that are naturally sweet, such as fresh or dried fruit, nuts and seeds, is a much healthier option. And go for Rooibosch (redbush) tea or relaxing herbal teas, rather than tea and coffee, which are high in caffeine and can make you jittery. See page 207 for how to deal with cravings.

Embrace change

View change as a natural, inevitable and exciting move forward, not a threat. This allows you to cope with whatever changes come your way.

Organize your time

Work out your priorities so you can efficiently use your time and energy. Make a realistic 'to do' list at the beginning of each day. Learn to say no to people - you don't have to agree to everything people ask you to do.

Get moving

One of the best stress-busters is physical exercise. Research shows that regular activity helps speed up the metabolism and encourages the release of endorphins, the body's own feel-good hormones which improve your mood, putting you in a better frame of mind for dealing with difficult situations.

Top 10 Stress-busters

1. Take a step back from stressful situations to give you a clearer perspective.

2. You can't always control circumstances, but you can choose how you react to them.

3. Include plenty of magnesium-rich foods in your diet, such as spinach, brazil nuts and walnuts. Magnesium supports the nervous system and has calming properties, helping tackle the tiredness caused by stress.

4. Take a strong multivitamin and mineral supplement, such as Gynovite, together with the herbs Valerian and Rhodiola, which help calm you down.

5. Share your worries with family and friends. Tell them how you feel and ask for their support.

6. Face up to your worries. Trying to distract yourself from problems will never solve them.

7. Learn to unwind through meditation or yoga.

8. Get plenty of sleep.

9. Try to get away occasionally, even it's only for a few days.

10. Find things to laugh about.

Survey Results

In 2004, Blackmores, the leading natural health food company, conducted a stress survey which revealed that women experience stress more than men, with most women suffering from stress at some point in their lives. The survey found that 47% of women feel there is too much to do and not enough time in the day, while 39% feel there is too much pressure placed on them to be everything to everyone. Managing household finances and grocery shopping are major causes of stress for 30% of women, while 45% feel flat and tired all the time and suffer from the effects of stress, including memory loss.

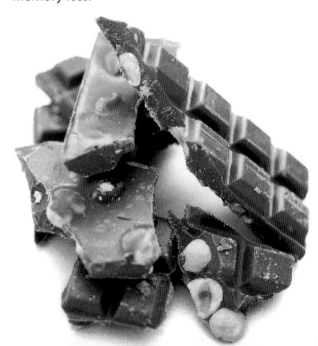

Blackmores' Survey Findings

Women's stress statistics:

- 73% of women suffer from stress at some point in their daily life.

- Women living in suburbia suffer the highest rates of stress (68%).

- Almost 40% of women suffer from stress on a regular basis. A further 59% of women suffer from occasional stress.

- 47% of women surveyed feel there is too much to do and not enough time in the day.

- 39% of women feel there is too much pressure placed on them to be everything to everyone.

- 30% of women find household finances and grocery shopping major causes of stress.

- 50% of women are more likely than men to use something or try something to deal with stress.

- 21% of women feel out of control of their lives.

- 45% of women feel tired all the time and suffer from the effects of stress and memory loss.

- 50% of women who are married or have a defacto partner suffer from stress.

- 41% of women suffer from stress when there are kids living at home.

46% of women suffering from stress are currently not working.

Did You Know?

According to the survey:

- 38% of women react to stress by eating chocolate.

- 29% argue or yell at someone.

- 24% have a cigarette.

- 23% get drunk.

- 47% take time out or talk to family or friends.

- Only 4% of women turn to yoga as a way of dealing with stress.

"Research shows that just 20 minutes of formal relaxation a day can reduce hot flashes by over 50%."

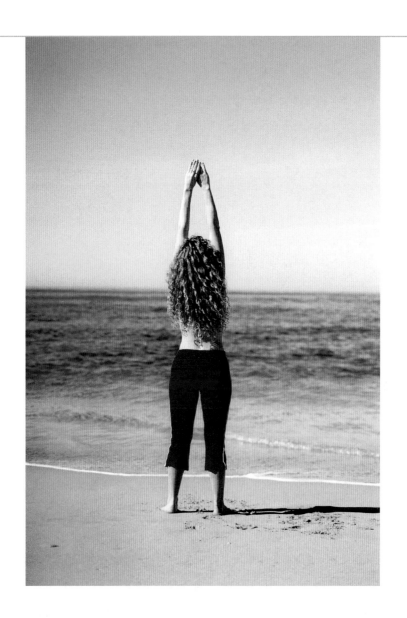

rest and relax

We saw in the previous chapter how too much stress can have a negative effect on your health and wellbeing, and more specifically can exacerbate symptoms such as hot flashes. Relaxation can have the exact opposite effect, but when you're tired and wound up, relaxing can be difficult, so you may need to explore more formal relaxation therapies to help relieve stress and associated anxiety.

If you find it difficult to relax as your mind remains active, it is a good idea to have pen and paper next to you so you can make a note of any important thoughts, allowing you to leave them behind as you move into your relaxation session. Relaxation is a practised art which takes time to develop. But once you have the art finely honed, you will be a much calmer person.

At the NHAS, we have found yoga, Pilates and creative visualization to be especially soothing.

"According to research, applied relaxation may be a good alternative to estrogen for treating hot flashes."

183

Yoga

Yoga has been practised throughout the world for thousands of years. It works on the principle that mind, body and soul need to be working in perfect harmony for optimal health. To help you achieve this, yoga uses asanas (postures that relax muscles) and pranayama (breathing techniques that help improve oxygen flow in your body and regulate your breathing). Meditation and relaxation exercises help to still the mind. It is best to attend a yoga class to learn the basic postures, then practise at home on a regular basis.

Pilates

Pilates is a more recent relaxation therapy that also exercises the body. Developed in the 1920s, this combination of Eastern and Western philosophies teaches you breathing techniques with movement, body mechanics, balance, co-ordination, positioning of the body, spatial awareness, strength and flexibility. As with yoga, you should first go to some classes to learn the moves before practising them at home.

When you're feeling anxious and tired, you sometimes need a hand to help you relax. Try Sue Fisher Hendry's 20-minute guided relaxation session on your *Get Fit For Midlife* DVD. Sue has been working with women for years, helping them to relax. Let her take you gently through the steps and feel yourself unwind and let go.

Creative Visualization

This simple, enjoyable way to relax requires little or no training and is ideal if you don't have enough time for yoga or Pilates. All you need to do is:

1. Lie flat on the floor with your head supported.

2. Bend your knees, keeping your feet flat on the floor (the Alexander lying position).

3. Close your eyes, breathe steadily and slowly, while consciously relaxing your face, fingers, arms, legs and toes.

4. Continue to breathe slowly and steadily. Start to visualize something you fancy, anything from a world cruise to a wonderful night out. The trick is to keep your mind focused on your fantasy for as long as you can. After 15-20 minutes, bring yourself gently back to reality, rolling onto your side before you stand up.

5. Creative visualization does require practice and you may have to work at it before you feel the full benefits. If your mind is very busy, it can help to jot down your thoughts in writing before you start so you can stay focused on your fantasy.

Did You Know?

15-20 minutes of relaxation a day can reduce hot flashes by up to 60%.

Learn to let go

Try this simple exercise to release muscle tension. It only takes 15-20 minutes. Once you've got the hang of it, you can do it anywhere at any time.

Get ready

Instead of focusing on the outside world and its problems, tune in to your body and become aware of your tension. Wear loose, comfortable clothes and find a warm, quiet place where you won't be interrupted. Put on some calming music to help you relax and adjust the lighting so you feel comfortable. Lie down on the floor or your bed.

Relax into it

1. Place a pillow beneath your head and relax your arms and lower jaw.

2. Take a few slow, deep breaths.

3. Concentrate on relaxing your muscles, starting with the toes on one foot, then on the other foot. Gradually work your way up your body.

4. Tense each group of muscles, then relax them, breathing deeply as you do so.

5. When you reach your head and your face feels relaxed, remain in this position for 15 minutes.

6. Gradually allow yourself to 'come to'. Roll onto your side, sit up slowly and sip a glass of water.

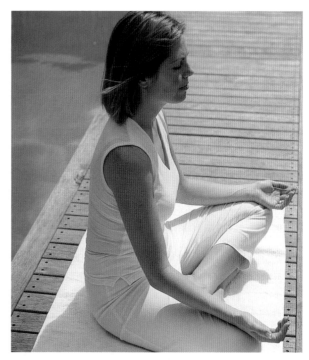

Research File

According to Swedish researchers, applied relaxation may be a good alternative to estrogen for treating hot flashes. In one study, 30 menopausal women suffering hot flashes were given either 12 weeks of estrogen treatment or applied relaxation. After three months, relaxation techniques had helped halve the number of hot flashes, and the flashes almost halved again after another three months. Estrogen worked faster, producing a 90% improvement within three months, helping women manage mood swings.

Relaxation and making time for yourself is important. If your sleep is constantly disrupted because of night sweats, it can be very wearing and frustrating. Enter the Pzizz program.

This power-napping tool combines several different proven techniques to give you the most refreshing and revitalising nap possible. It is a blend of Neuro Linguistic Programming with specially composed music, sound effects and a beat that induces a wonderfully relaxed state. You can vary the length of the session and create a tailor-made program.

You can listen to it via your computer or download the programs onto your iPod or MP3 player so you can take it with you wherever you go. I often use mine after a hard day's work before going out in the evening. Just 20 minutes with my Pzizz programme gives me the same feeling as a two-hour nap.

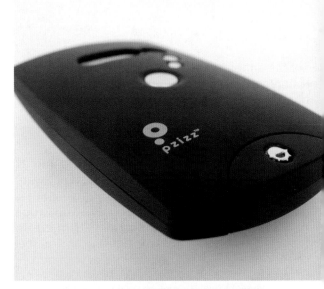

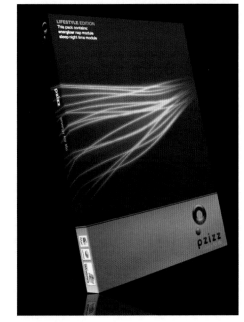

I felt exhausted by my symptoms as they kept me awake at night. I found it incredibly difficult to relax due to being so stressed at work. Maryon gave me a lot of good advice about my diet and suggested I take a series of supplements to help, and they did.

Dealing with my work stress took some time. We implemented a plan to get me more in control of my time at work, and I began using the Pzizz machine at lunch time to help me relax and rest. I found this enormously helpful and I really do feel like I have had a restful sleep, even after only 20 minutes of using the Pzizz program. I carry it around with me and wouldn't be without it now.

These days I am pretty much symptom free, I feel so much more relaxed and energized and look forward to my days with confidence.

Betty Evans

notes

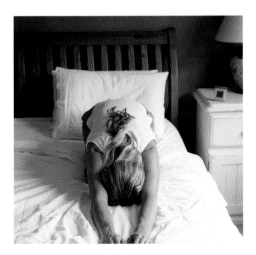

"This is such a good time, because we can still be sexy."

Diana Moran

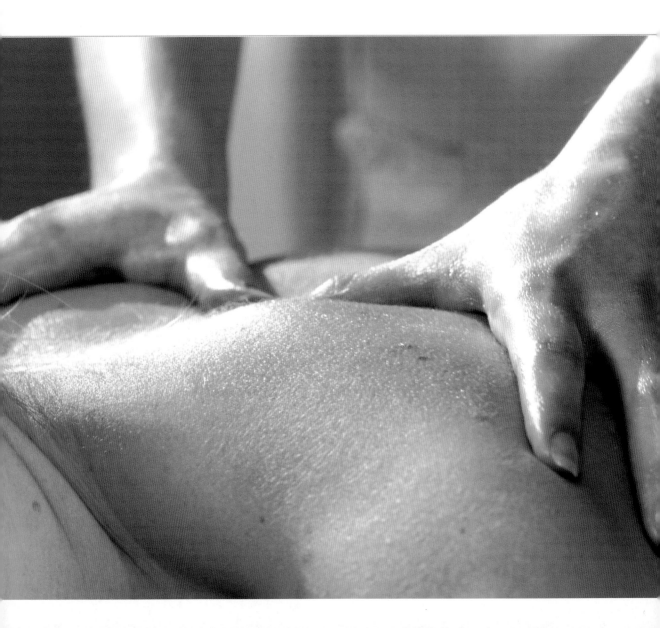

alternatively speaking

By the time you reach menopause, problems associated with not meeting your nutritional needs at various stages in life, being pregnant and breastfeeding, coping with stressful situations and perhaps suffering premenstrual symptoms, may well have stacked the cards against you. Following our Natural Menopause Program will definitely help put you back in the driver's seat of life. If you need an extra boost, complementary therapies can help bring relief from certain symptoms.

The stresses and strains of life can leave us feeling twisted, knotted and out of sorts. I often find that particular complementary therapies work very well alongside our program. For example, neck and back pain respond well to cranial osteopathy and acupuncture. Homeopathy and herbal medicine can also help acute symptoms in the short-term.

"Fourteen per cent of the women in our Midlife Survey tried homoeopathy, of whom seventy six per cent found it helpful."

Herbal Medicine

Herbal medicine has been used for thousands of years to help treat common conditions. Many herbs have now undergone clinical trials to examine how they work and why, and we have incorporated more herbal medicine into our program. The most tried and tested herbs to help combat symptoms of menopause are red clover, ginseng, St John's Wort, sage, Dong Quai, valerian and vitex agnus castus. Twenty four per cent of the women in our Midlife Survey had tried herbs, of whom 80% found them useful.

Acupuncture and Acupressure

Many problems that occur at the time of menopause may respond to acupuncture. This treatment uses fine needles inserted at specific points in your body, known as meridians, to help unblock energy channels. It is not uncommon for energy in the body to become blocked, leading to all manner of symptoms from irritability and anxiety to insomnia and headaches.

Acupressure, which involves applying pressure at certain points on your body with your fingertips, can also be a useful self-help tool. Nine per cent of the women in our Midlife Survey tried a course of acupuncture, of whom 74% found it helpful.

Homoeopathy

Whereas conventional medicine aims to treat people with a drug, homoeopathy was developed to treat like with like. The word homoeopathy comes from the Greek 'homoeo' (meaning similar) and 'pathos' (meaning suffering). It is designed to produce the same symptoms from which you are suffering. This is said to stimulate the body to fight back against them. The dosages are very small and often only contain an energy or 'spirit' of the original medicine.

Sepia and sulphur are two of the many remedies that may be indicated for hot flashes and night sweats. There is also a wide choice of remedies for poor memory, depression, insomnia, anxiety attacks, irritability, headaches and confusion.

Fourteen per cent of the women in our Midlife Survey tried homoeopathy, of whom 76% found it helpful.

"Soon after I started on Maryon's program, I hurt my back and went to see an acupuncturist. It seemed to have a calming effect and complemented the program very well."
Cherie Lunghi

Cranial Osteopathy

Cranial osteopathy involves gentle manipulation of the body's soft tissues. It can also help with long-standing back, head and neck problems, and it has been shown to reduce hot flashes. Treatment for women suffering menopausal symptoms is often aimed at improving function of the pituitary gland. This gland, found at the base of the brain, balances the function of the adrenal glands and consequently many of the body's functions.

Watch Point

Whichever complementary therapy you go for, it is important to put yourself in the hands of an experienced and qualified practitioner. These days, the more recognized complementary specialities have official associations that keep registers of qualified practitioners. You can contact these practitioners locally or ask for a recommendation in your local health store.

Research File

Several small studies have suggested that homoeopathy may help women with menopausal symptoms, including hot flashes, fatigue and mood disturbances. However, more research is required to accurately determine how beneficial homoeopathy really is.

notes

"A lot of women at the time of menopause are worried about osteoporosis and are keen to improve their health for the long-term future."

Dr Sally Hope

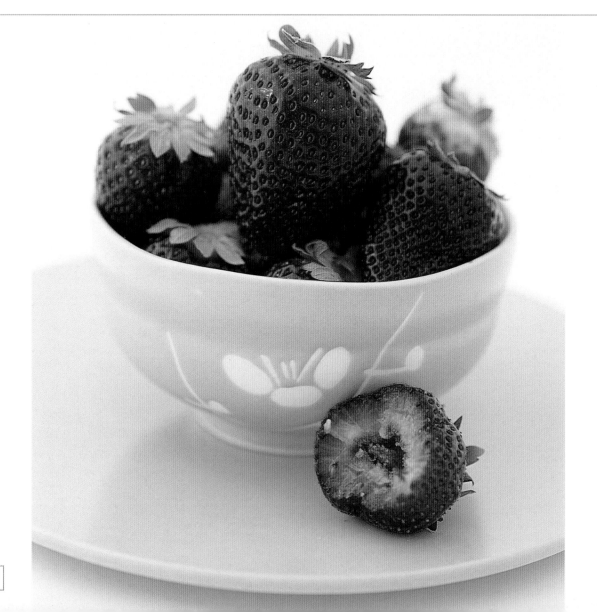

boost your nutrient levels

The menopause is often a time when nutritional deficiencies start to become apparent. A combination of years of wear and tear, pregnancy and breastfeeding can all challenge our nutrient stores, while our lack of knowledge of how to replace what time and nature have taken away leaves many of us in a nutritionally depleted state, which can affect our brain chemistry and our hormonal balance.

We know from previous chapters that women of childbearing age can have low levels of important nutrients, which plays havoc with their cycle. To make matters worse, some of these important nutrients become in even shorter supply as we age, so by the time we get to perimenopause, it becomes almost impossible for many women not to experience raging hormones.

You may think your diet is healthy, but if you start to analyse it more closely, a different story might emerge. A few years ago, a group of staff at National Magazines completed the following questionnaire for me about their diet, as well as a questionnaire that assessed whether they were in good nutritional shape. Not one of the participants was consuming an adequate diet and all had some signs of nutritional deficiencies. We are all in the same boat, as we generally lack knowledge about how to meet the nutritional needs of our body.

Is Your Diet Good for You?

Circle the box most relevant to your consumption in each of these 30 categories:

Food	Optimum	Questionable	Really Bad
Cows' milk (full cream, reduced fat (2%) and non-fat)	2 litres or more per week	1-2 litres per week (unless on exclusion diet and replaced by soy milk)	less than 1 litre per week (unless on exclusion diet and replaced by soy milk)
Soy milk (calcium-fortified)	2 litres or more per week	1-2 litres per week	less than 1 litre per week
Cheese (full fat or reduced fat)	125-250g per week	50-124g per week	0-49g per week
Eggs	3-6 per week	1-2 per week	none
Main meal with protein (animal or vegetable)	Every day	5 or 6 per week	4 or less per week
Breakfast	Every day	5 or 6 per week	4 or less per week
Fruits, vegetables and salad	5 or more servings per day	3-4 servings per day	2 servings or less per day
Butter	25g or less per week	26-50g per week	more than 50g per week
White bread	None per day	1-2 slices per day	3 or more slices per day
Wholegrain bread	2-3 slices per day	1 slice per day	none (unless wheat-free diet)
Vegetable oil	1 tsp per day	2 tsp -1 tbsp per day	more than 1 tbsp per day

Food	Optimum	Questionable	Really Bad
Hard margarine	none	up to 25g per week	more than 25g per week
Glasses of water	6 or more per day	3-5 per day	less than 3 per day
Cups of tea or coffee	0-2 per day	3-5 per day	6 or more per day
Alcoholic drinks	7 per week (less than 10 units per week)	8-14 per week (11-20 units)	15 per week (21 units or more)
Cola-based drinks (non-diet and diet)	0-1 per week	2-3 per week	4 or more per week
Chocolate bars or equivalent	0-1 per week	2-3 per week	4 or more per week
Cookies	0-4 per week	5-14 per week	15 or more per week
Cakes and puddings	0-2 per week	3-5 per week	6 or more per week
Candy	0-1 per day	2-3 per day	4 or more per day
Teaspoons of sugar added to each tea or coffee	none	1/2 - 1	1 or more
Servings of pizza or white pasta	0-1 per week	2-3 per week	4 or more per week
Packets of chips	0-1 per week	2-3 per week	4 or more per week
Salt added to food	never	occasionally	regularly

Food	Optimum	Questionable	Really Bad
Servings of fish	2 or more per week	1 per week	never
Portions of lean red meat	3 per week	less than 2 or more than 5 per week	0-1 per week unless a vegetarian
Servings of sausages, bacon or pies	0-3 per week	4-5 per week	6 or more per week
Fast food (burger, pizza, Chinese, Mexican, fried chicken, fish and fries etc)	0-1 per week	2 per week	3 or more per week
Servings of fresh potatoes (not French fries)	4 or more per week	2-3 per week	0-1 per week
Skip a meal	never	1-2 per week	3 or more per week

Your Scores

• If you circled 25 or more in the Optimum column, you are doing really well with your diet.

• If you circled 18-24 in the Optimum column, you're not doing badly, but there is room for improvement.

• If you circled 17 or less in the Optimum column, and circled everything else in the Questionable column, you need to improve your eating habits. Your nutritional state could be exacerbating menopausal symptoms, as well as other menopause-related problems, especially osteoporosis.

(Write your scores down in the notes section of your Natural Menopause Plan on page 322. Repeat this questionnaire again in four month's time and compare your scores).

The good news is that the Natural Menopause Program can help you get back on the right track, so get started with our diet Do's and Don'ts. Your goal is to restore estrogen levels and put back some of the nutrients that time and nature have removed, including magnesium, zinc, B vitamins and essential fatty acids.

DO

1. Include at least 100mg of phytoestrogen in your daily diet, spread throughout the day to satisfy the needs of the estrogen receptor sites. Best sources include soy products, linseeds and red clover. Other lesser sources can be found in chickpeas, lentils, mung beans, alfalfa, sunflower seeds, pumpkin seeds, sesame seeds, rhubarb and green and yellow vegetables. Golden flaxseeds are also rich in phytoestrogen and can be added to breakfast cereals. They are also a good source of fiber and can help constipation.

2. Have a total of five servings of fresh fruits and vegetables per day. These provide plenty of potassium and magnesium, plus small amounts of phytoestrogen. Where possible, eat organic products or grow your own.

3. Go for foods rich in calcium and magnesium, such as milk, green leafy vegetables, unsalted nuts and seeds, wholegrains and bony fish, including sardines and trout.

4. Eat regularly. Three meals a day help to ensure a good balanced diet, as well as a steady flow of energy throughout the day.

5. Include enough protein from animal or vegetarian sources in at least one meal a day. Low-protein diets jeopardise the balance of many nutrients, including calcium, Vitamin B and iron.

6. Limit your consumption of red meat to one or two portions a week. Go for fish, poultry, peas, beans and nuts instead.

7. Add two tablespoons of Golden Roasted Flaxseeds to your daily breakfast cereal, yogurt or fruit salad. This is an easy way to get another 'phyto fix' during the day. Flaxseeds are one of the richest sources of natural phytoestrogen and are also a good source of fiber, which can help alleviate constipation.

8. Have a serving of dairy products each day. This may be milk added to cereal or drinks, cheese or yogurt. These provide calcium and additional amounts of protein. Go for low-fat options if you need to lose weight, but avoid fully non-fat milk, which contains no Vitamin A (2% is preferable).

9. Drink plenty of liquids, preferably the equivalent of at least six glasses of water daily, which can include herbal and fruit tea. Redbush or Tick Tock tea can be made with milk and makes a good alternative to ordinary tea, but remember to let your hot drinks cool down as the hot water may bring on a flash.

10. Consume three portions of oily fish per week, including salmon, mackerel, herring, or sardines, which are a rich source of omega-3 and help with hormone health, as well as healthy joints.

11. Keep a supply of nutritious snacks to eat between meals if you get hungry. Nuts, Phyto Fix Bars (see recipes), unsalted nuts and seeds, fresh fruit or dried fruit that hasn't been dipped in sulphur dioxide are ideal.

12. Consider taking some of the recommended nutritional supplements to help boost your nutrient levels in the short-term.

Don't

1. Go overboard on alcohol. Limit yourself to three drinks per week or less. Alcohol aggravates flashes, insomnia and, in excess, can worsen or cause many nutritional deficiencies at a time when you need to be conserving essential nutrients.

2. Drink endless cups of coffee and tea. Caffeine can aggravate flashes, as well as anxiety and insomnia, so go for herbal alternatives instead.

3. Go for curry or other heavily spiced food as the hot spices, like hot drinks and alcohol, can bring on the power surges.

4. Eat sugar and junk food, including sugar added to tea and coffee, sweets, cakes, cookies, chocolate, jam, puddings, marmalade, honey, ice cream and soft drinks containing phosphates. Consumption of these may reduce the uptake of essential nutrients and cause water retention and bloating.

5. Add salt to your cooking or at the table, as we already have far more salt than we need from hidden sources. Avoid salted foods like kippers and bacon. Salt causes fluid retention and encourages calcium loss from the body in your urine. Use potassium-rich salt substitutes or other flavorings such as garlic, onion, kelp powder, fresh herbs, sesame powder or other mild spices.

6. Eat foods containing wheat and bran, in the short-term, if you feel bloated or experience wind or constipation.

7. Eat lots of fatty food. Aim to limit your intake of fats to no more than 30% of your dietary intake. For most of us, this means reducing consumption by at least 25%. Avoid hydrogenated fats and anything other than small amounts of butter. Instead go for the cold-pressed oils, including sunflower, sesame, safflower, as well as olive oil.

8. Light up after a meal, as smoking cigarettes can aggravate hot flashes and night sweats and can bring on an earlier menopause. If you do smoke, try to pace yourself between cigarettes and cut down gradually until you can manage to quit the habit altogether.

9. Finally, don't go shopping on an empty stomach otherwise you may be tempted to fill your basket with those high-fat, calorie-laden foods you are supposed to be avoiding.

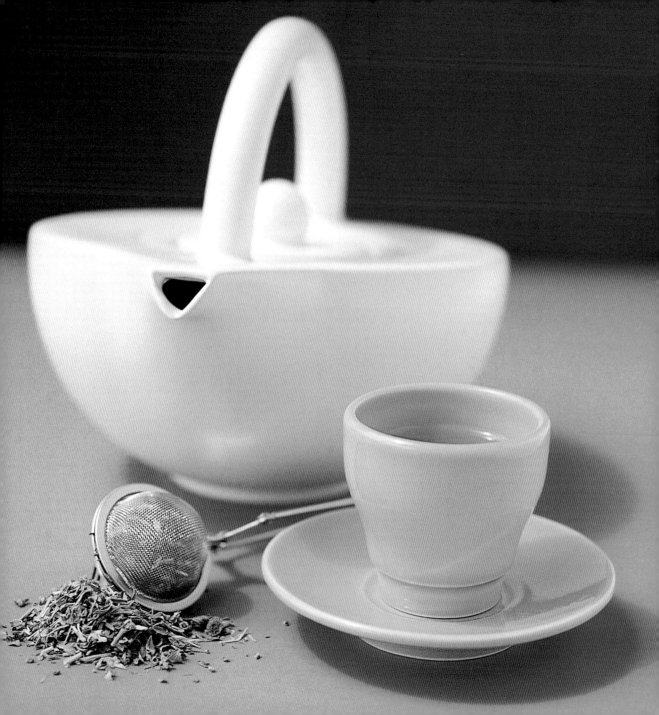

"People now comment on how great my skin looks, which has boosted my confidence and made me feel so much better."

Sarah Adams

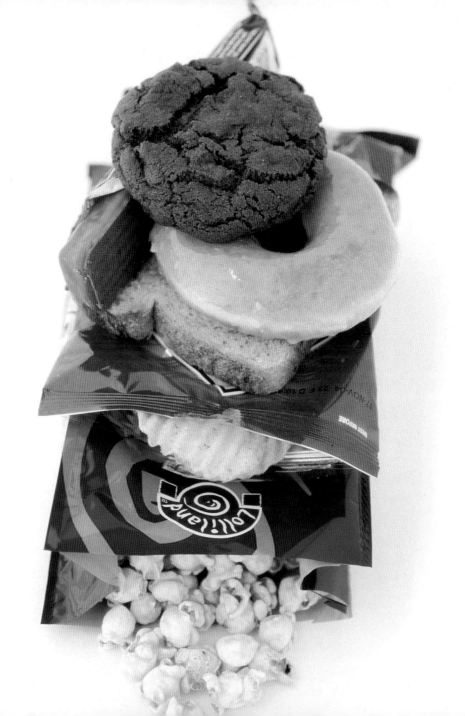

coping with cravings

Craving food, particularly chocolate, is very common. It affects a staggering 75% of women in the USA to some degree, with 40% admitting that chocolate is their problem. The bad news is that these cravings can get worse around the time of menopause. And it's often the cravings getting the better of us that causes us to pile on the pounds and subsequently find it impossible to lose that extra weight.

Interestingly, there is often a physiological reason for cravings. The brain and nervous system require a constant supply of good nutrients in order to function normally, but our stressful lives mean that we don't always eat as healthily as we should. We skip meals or eat on the run. As a result, our blood-sugar levels drop and we start to crave a glucose fix to give us energy.

So what do we do? We grab the nearest bar of chocolate or cookie, which may give us a quick surge of glucose-fuelled energy, but is hardly nutritious. What's more, this quick energy buzz is usually temporary, so before too long we're craving something sweet again and so the cycle continues, playing havoc with our waistlines.

The trick is to know how to break this cycle, which often develops into a real addiction and, just like alcohol, drugs, smoking, or other habits, this involves a period of withdrawal.

Do food cravings have a hold over you?

Answer Yes or No to the following questions:

	Yes	No		Yes	No
Are you embarrassed about the amount of chocolate and sweet cookies you consume?	☐	☐	If you don't have chocolate at home, do you sometimes go out especially to buy some?	☐	☐
Do you graze on chocolate, cookies and chips, etc throughout the day?	☐	☐	Do you eat cookies, cake, fruit pies, desserts or other food containing sugar most days?	☐	☐
Do you make impulse purchases of junk food?	☐	☐	Do you eat more than 3 bars of chocolate per week?	☐	☐
Do you take sugar in your tea or coffee?	☐	☐	Have you ever bought chocolate as a gift, then eaten it yourself?	☐	☐
Do you drink more than 3 soft drinks per week?	☐	☐	Do you regularly consume ice cream?	☐	☐
Do you routinely eat sweet food after meals or in the evening?	☐	☐	Do you crave salty food like chips, salted nuts, Marmite or soy sauce?	☐	☐
Have you been guilty of eating the children's chocolate or treats?	☐	☐	Do you feel hooked on certain types of food?	☐	☐
Do you prefer chocolate to sex?	☐	☐	Have you ever eaten chocolate and hidden the wrappers so that no one else knows?	☐	☐
Do you have a stash of comfort food?	☐	☐			

If you answered Yes to three or more of these questions, you need to take some action. Five Yes checks means things are out of your control and over six means you're a chocoholic! But there is a solution, so don't panic. Enter your score on your Natural Menopause Plan on page 322.

Action Plan

When it comes to controlling your cravings, it is important to monitor what you eat and when you eat it. You will be amazed how giving your diet an overhaul and making a few tweaks can help keep your blood glucose levels on an even keel, which means you're not always longing for your next chocolate fix. As a result, any excess weight will drop off. Here are some goals to aim for:

- Consume nutritious food - little and often - to keep blood-sugar levels constant. Eat breakfast, lunch and dinner every day, with a wholesome mid-morning and mid-afternoon snack.

- Eat fresh, home-cooked, nutritious foods whenever possible.

- Eat foods that are intrinsically sweet, like dried fruit, fresh fruit, nuts and seeds.

- Relax while you're eating and enjoy your food.

- Plan your meals and snacks in advance (bearing in mind that calorie requirements are increased by up to 500 calories per day during the premenstrual week for women).

- Always shop for food after you have eaten, not when you are hungry.

- Cut down on tea and coffee. If these are consumed in large amounts, they can cause an increase in the release of insulin. Large amounts of sugar consumed in tea or coffee can also contribute to an unstable blood glucose level. Try Rooiboos (or Redbush) tea, which is a herbal tea look-alike, or coffee substitutes that are available in health food shops.

- Concentrate on a diet rich in chromium, magnesium and Vitamins B and C, including whole grains, chili, black pepper, chicken and peppers.

- Reduce your intake of alcohol. Apart from the fact that alcohol is high in calories, in excess it can cause liver damage, which can lead to significant hypoglycaemia or low blood sugar. Replacing a meal with two or three gin and tonics, for example, can cause a profound rise and subsequent fall in blood glucose levels, producing all the symptoms of hypoglycaemia (low blood sugar).

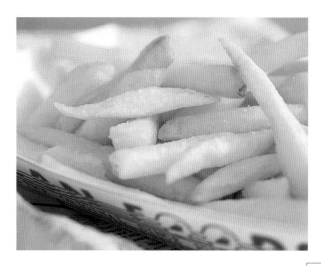

Craving Saviors

Making sure you are getting enough of the right nutrients to keep your blood glucose at optimum levels is the key to beating your cravings. Essential nutrients for regulating blood sugar are the B vitamins (necessary for optimum function of the brain and the nervous system), magnesium (necessary for normal hormone function) and the trace element chromium.

We are born with only one sixteenth of an ounce of the trace mineral chromium and it gets less as we age. Magnesium is the most common deficiency among women and B vitamins are often in short supply. All of these important nutrients are necessary for normal blood glucose control helping to keep our cravings at bay.

The B vitamins, magnesium and chromium can be sourced in food, but you have to know where to look for them (see page 88). You may also want to consider taking a specially formulated nutritional supplement that acts as a short-term nutritional prop to regulate blood-sugar levels. For example, a chromium supplement that contains B vitamins and magnesium, as well as a little Vitamin C, are available through our website www.askmaryonstewart.com/member or our Mail Order Service (see page 370).

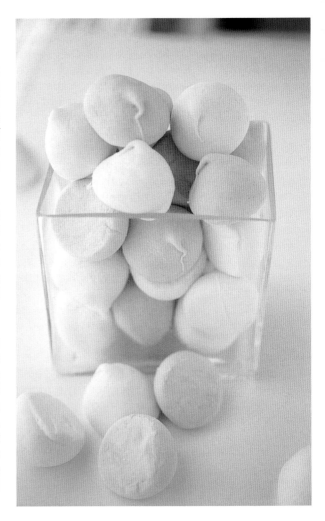

Eleanor's Story

Eleanor Burns, 53, had been on HRT for six months. When she started to put on weight, she decided to look for a natural alternative.

I took HRT for six months, but due to weight gain and general feelings of compromised health, I decided to go down the alternative route. Here's Health magazine wrote an article entitled 'Natural help for the menopause', which caught my attention. The article explained how menopause can be controlled by making dietary modifications and taking herbal and nutritional supplements. It made reference to the NHAS, so I contacted Maryon Stewart and made an appointment to see her at the London clinic.

After my initial consultation, Maryon recommended dietary modifications, some exercise, relaxation and nutritional supplements. After just four weeks of closely following the recommendations, my health improved and I even lost weight! I wasn't used to eating legumes and tofu, so Maryon suggested I read The Phyto Factor, which explains how you can incorporate phytoestrogen into your daily diet with ease. The recipe and menu section was excellent and I soon got to work in the kitchen!

The difference in my symptoms now is quite remarkable. The flashes, loss of libido and general fatigue, which were moderately to severely problematic, are now mild to non-existent.

"Making sure you are getting enough of the right nutrients to keep your blood glucose at optimum levels is key if you want to beat your cravings."

"Menopause is an excellent time to take stock of the rest of your life, because at menopause you may only be half way there."

Susan Wysocki

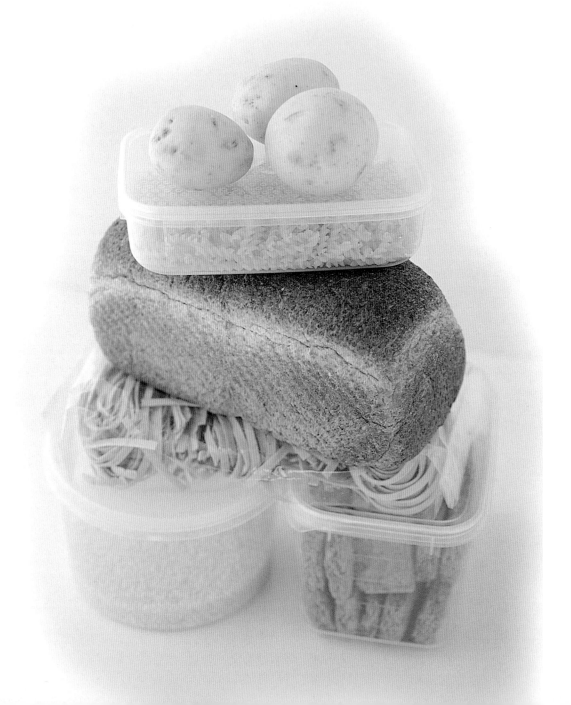

beat the bloat

At the time of menopause, our nutrient levels often become unacceptably low. As a result, our immune system, which protects us from toxins, often struggles to work efficiently.

Our impaired immune system perceives certain foods and drinks as 'toxic', leading to all manner of symptoms. Irritability, anxiety, constipation, abdominal bloating, dairrhea, excessive gas, irritable bowel, fatigue, depression and even insomnia can be aggravated by eating these 'toxic' foods. The good news is that these conditions can usually be reversed over a few months by improving our nutrient levels.

Transient food sensitivities cause many women to produce antibodies to some foods and drinks. This process can result in water retention, as the brain instructs the cells to retain fluid in an attempt to dilute the so-called 'toxins'. The most common temporary sensitivity is to whole wheat and grains, such as wheat, oats, barley, rye and bran. When these are excluded from your diet for a month or two, it can lead to rapid weight loss as the redundant fluid is passed.

Is Food the Culprit?

Start by answering Yes or No to the following questions to see if you have a food sensitivity:

	Yes	No
Do you suffer from constipation?	☐	☐
Do you feel bloated after eating?	☐	☐
Do you suffer from excessive wind?	☐	☐
Is dairrhea a problem?	☐	☐
Do you feel tired and depressed?	☐	☐
Do you feel anxious for no apparent reason?	☐	☐
Do you suffer from IBS?	☐	☐

If you answered Yes to more than two of these questions, you may have developed a temporary intolerance to grains, in which case you should aim to cut them out of your diet for a while. Our Action Plan below will help get you going. Don't forget to enter your score in your Natural Menopause Plan on page 322.

Action Plan

Cut Them Out

Stop eating wheat, oats, barley, rye and bran for at least four weeks, preferably for six weeks. Most supermarkets and health food stores sell a wide range of wheat-free breads, crackers, pasta, pizza bases, muffins, cakes and cookies.

After four to six weeks, if you feel your symptoms have improved, you can start to reintroduce the various grains one by one back into your diet. For example, choose one grain, such as rye in the form of Ryvita crackers. If you have no reaction after five days, choose another grain and repeat the process. Don't mix the grains because if you get a reaction, you won't know which grain caused the reaction. It is best to try wheat last, as this grain causes the most problems.

Typical reactions include:

• Dairrhea or constipation
• Excessive gas and abdominal bloating
• Headaches and irritability
• Weight gain
• Confusion
• Depression
• Mouth ulcers
• Skin rash
• Palpitations

Is it For Ever?

If you get a reaction to a grain, try to establish what you have reacted to and avoid eating it for a month or two before trying to reintroduce it again. Wait until your body settles down, then try introducing another grain.

There is a distinction between 'food sensitivity' and 'food allergy'. We often find that severe menopause symptoms are caused by food sensitivities, rather than an actual food allergy.

A small number of women discover they have a permanent allergy to a particular food and soon realise they are better off avoiding that food altogether, rather than suffering unnecessarily.

If your symptoms are severe, it is a good idea to give your body a complete rest for at least two or three months. It can take as long as six months, or even a year, for your body to get back to normal and learn to cope again with foods that were previously eliminated.

Foods Containing Grains

A huge number of the foods we commonly eat contain grains. To get an idea of how prevalent grains are in our foods, next time you're in the supermarket, have a closer look at some of the labels. You may be surprised by what you find!

Wheat

The most obvious foods containing wheat include bread, cookies, cakes, pasta, cereals, pastries and flour made from wheat and other ingredients.

Wheat is often found in prepared sauces, soups and processed foods such as sausages.

If you are on a wheat-free diet, it is recommended that you also avoid gluten-free products, as some of these still contain wheat. Wheat is sometimes disguised as modified starch, rusk and cereal filler.

Oats

These are usually found in porridge, oat cookies, flapjacks and oat flakes.

Rye

This is found in rye bread (which may also contain wheat), pumpernickel and Ryvita crackers.

Barley

This is often found in tinned or packet soups, as well as barley drinks.

"As the months passed, I felt happier and more positive than I had for years. The weight started to fall off... Now I feel calm and happy to the point of feeling bubbly."

Jo De Lisle

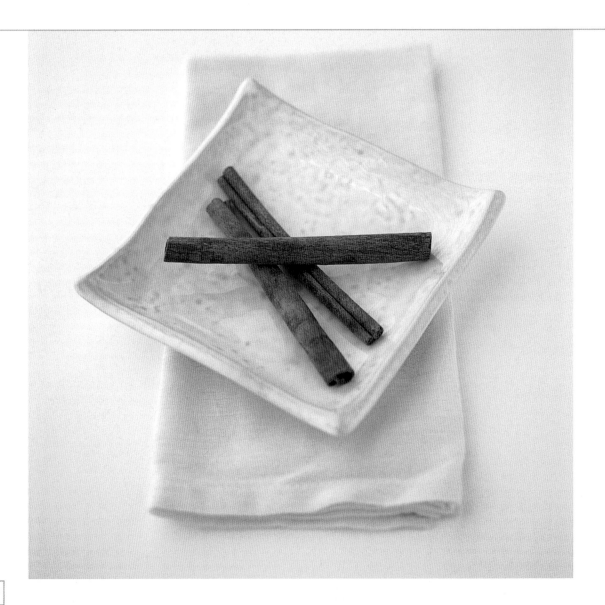

supplementary benefits

However healthily you eat, sometimes it just isn't possible to achieve the desired balance of nutrients through diet alone, but you can easily make up for any shortfall with a selection of carefully chosen supplements.

Our Natural Menopause Program recommends standardized supplements that have undergone properly conducted clinical trials. It is vitally important to choose a supplement that has been standardized and has had the isoflavone content verified independently. (Unfortunately, the isoflavone content of many isoflavone-rich supplements varies considerably from that stated on the label).

Depending on your symptoms, there are several useful supplements that you can try in conjunction with each other. Most of these are available online at www.askmaryonstewart.com/member or in pharmacies and health food stores.

The best option is to take a multivitamin and mineral supplement that contains good amounts of the essential nutrients mentioned.

Gynovite

We recommend Gynovite, which was formulated by a professor of obstetrics and gynaecology in the US especially for women from menopause onwards. Clinical trials have found that it helps get nutrient levels back into an optimum range, thus improving hormone balance and bone density. Another good choice is Swiss One "10" Classic Multi, a similar formulation tailored for the Canadian market. They are available by mail order (see page 370 or at www.askmaryonstewart.com/member.

Isoflavone-Rich Supplements

If your symptoms are severe, a combination of a phyto-rich diet and isoflavone-rich supplements can bring the best results in the shortest time.

Promensil

Over the past six years, we have used the isoflavone-rich supplement Promensil, which is a standardized red clover product made by the Australian company, Novogen. It contains high concentrations of the isoflavones genistein, daidzein, formononetin and biochanin. Red clover is the richest known source of these four estrogenic isoflavones. It has up to 10 times as much of these isoflavones as the next richest source, soy. Each 500mg tablet of Promensil is designed to deliver the same dose of isoflavones as a vegetarian diet based on legumes (approximately 40mg of the four isoflavones). Taking Promensil is the only way you are likely to get an adequate amount, especially if you don't digest soy products very well.

Cardiozen

Fish oils have been the subject of many clinical trials and proven to help relieve joint pain. Cardiozen is the fish oil supplement we use in our program as it is made from wholesome oil free of pollutants. And in case you are worried that it might taste of fish, the oil is processed in such a way that it has a minimal fishy after taste or smell. It also contains co-enzyme Q10, which is important for muscle energy. In addition, CoQ10 can safeguard against deficiencies which can be caused by statins. Cardiozen contains more than 80% of omega-3 fatty acids, of which at least 50% is the important EPA. Just one capsule a day will address most people's requirements for this crucial, and very beneficial nutrient.

Phyto Soy

There are many soy isoflavone supplements on the market, but they vary in quality. Phyto Soya capsules, produced by Arkopharma, are standardised and come in two strengths (17.5mg and 35mg of isoflavones per capsule). In an abstract of a forthcoming medical paper presented at the North American Menopause Society in October 2006 it stated that there were no adverse effects on the lining of the uterus in women taking this supplement for one year.

Phyto Soya Vaginal Gel

Until recently, the only solution for a dry vagina and pain during sex was a lubricating cream or an oestrogen cream. We now recommend Arkopharma's Phyto Soya Vaginal Gel, which is inserted in the vagina twice a week. This has been a great relief for many women on the programme.

Omega-7

Another product helping vaginal dryness that has recently undergone a positive trial in Denmark is Omega-7 by PharmaNord. Derived from Sea Buckthorn, a berry bush naturally found in Asia and Europe, results show it helps maintain the health and integrity of the mucous membranes in the vagina. Omega-7 has been used in Asian traditional medicine for over 1,000 years.

The seed oil contains omega-6 and omega-3, while the oil from the plant flesh is one of the few rich sources of omega-7 essential fatty acids (EFAs). For women experiencing severe vaginal dryness or bleeding during sex, we recommend two capsules of PharmaNord's Omega-7 in the morning and two in the evening. You'll be delighted with the results.

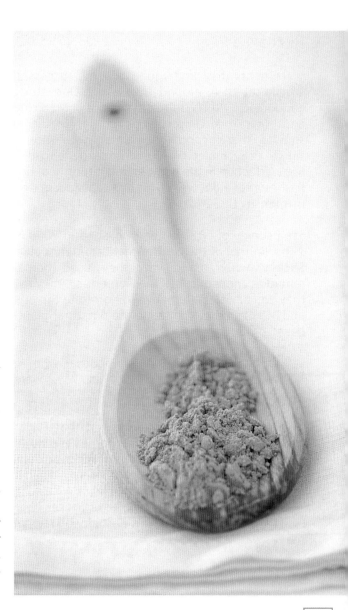

Research File

Promensil has undergone several successful clinical trials around the world. One study conducted by Tufts University School of Medicine and New York University School of Medicine showed that menopausal women who took a single daily tablet of Promensil experienced a 56% reduction in the number and intensity of hot flashes after eight weeks. Night sweats decreased in intensity by 52%.

In a survey of 781 women published in 2006 in The Journal of the North American Menopause Society, when asked why they used herbal remedies, more than half the women said they felt they were a safer alternative to hormone therapy and 45% said they wanted to use a 'natural' plant-based product.

Our own study of 100 menopausal women taking Promensil showed that 75% were symptom-free within four months.

A clinical trial carried out showed that Phyto Soy capsules can reduce hot flashes and other bothersome symptoms such as insomnia, anxiety, mood problems and loss of libido.

Clinical trials show that Phyto Soya Gel can help rehydrate and restore the elasticity of vaginal tissues within three weeks.

Promensil has been shown to help reverse vaginal atrophy. It does not cause thickening of the lining of the womb or have an adverse effect on breast tissue, a complication commonly associated with HRT. Also, no weight gain has been seen with Promensil, unlike HRT, which NHAS surveys have shown adds, on average, 8kg in the first year.

Why Supplement?

By using scientifically based supplements in addition to dietary changes, we can control hot flashes and night sweats much faster than by relying on diet alone. Before we used these estrogen-moderating supplements in our program, it used to take at least three or four months to control hot flashes. Once we included them, women began returning for their follow-up appointment within one month of their initial consultation, delighted that both their hot flashes and night sweats were far milder.

Once you have chosen your basic supplement, you need to add other appropriate products. Use the chart on page 228 to help decide which extra supplements you need. The supplements listed can also be ordered through our website www.askmaryonstewart.com/member or by calling us on 020 7107 0698.

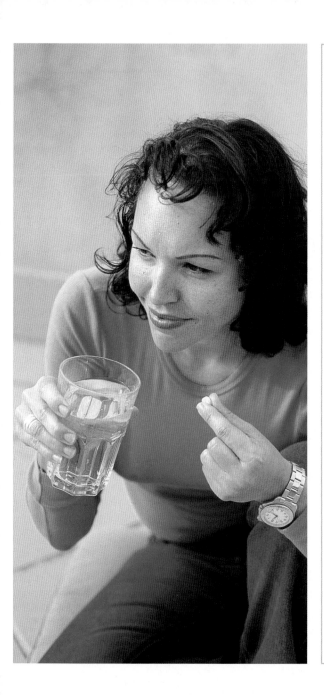

When and How to Take Your Supplements

Always start by taking your supplements gradually. For example, if it is recommended you take two to four capsules of a supplement per day, start by taking one tablet per day and gradually build up to the optimum dose over a week or two. Supplements should always be taken after meals, unless otherwise specified. If you are taking prescribed drugs from your doctor, do not reduce the dose without your doctor's agreement. Most of the supplements suggested here are compatible with medication. In fact, you may feel you have less need for medication. If you are taking prescribed drugs, check with your doctor before taking St John's Wort.

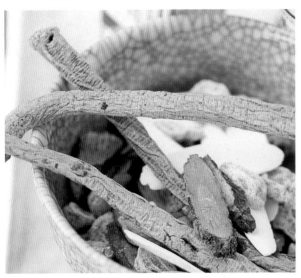

What About the Long-Term?

How long you continue to take your supplements is up to you. Supplements that are being taken to address certain symptoms can be reduced gradually once the symptoms are under control. If you reduce them too quickly and the symptoms return, you can always increase the dosage again.

You are most at risk of bone loss during the first five years after menopause. Although bone loss slows down in the following 10 years, it is still quite significant. So if you are at risk of osteoporosis, you may need to take supplements for some time, while also having a bone density scan every few years to check your bone mass.

Whether you continue to take isoflavone-rich supplements depends on the amount of isoflavones you have in your diet. Those who enjoy eating soy and settle into a routine will require less isoflavone-rich supplements in the long-term. Research now suggests that it is advisable to continue with an isoflavone-rich regime for the rest of your days to protect your bones, heart and cognitive function.

Jennifer's Story

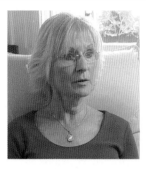

Jennifer Colby, a 51-year-old mother and post-mistress from Sussex, had been suffering with hot flashes and quite severe symptoms of arthritis for three years when she contacted me for advice.

When I was 48, my periods came to an end after only slight disruption and I thought I had escaped lightly. I had always been quite active and aware of what I ate and drank, so I assumed I had passed through menopause unscathed.

Then one day, the hot flashes suddenly arrived, taking me completely by surprise. I would get so hot I could smell my hair, and my heart would pound. Then they would subside, leaving me shivering and soaked with perspiration. It wasn't long before the night sweats began, several times a night, leaving me awake and fretful over the silliest things. I became very irritable and short-tempered and was constantly tired.

I read an article in Essentials magazine about the NHAS that recommended Maryon Stewart's book on menopause. I bought the book and read it,
not dreaming for a moment that I would one day become a Case History in it! I followed the self-help recommendations, adjusting my eating and drinking habits, and within weeks saw an improvement. Over several months, the severe day flashes reduced to milder sweats. The night sweats continued, but I was sleeping a little better.*

Then I started to feel pain in my thumb and finger joints, and they started to swell up. I also started to feel pain in my feet. The pain gradually became worse until I reached a point where holding a pen was unbearable.

Although I'd been following the diet recommended in the book, I had not taken any supplements, so I decided to contact the NHAS for advice. I was given a nutrition and exercise program and was advised to take Gynovite, Promensil and Cardiozen. After only a few weeks, the pains in my hands and feet had reduced dramatically and the flashes were slowly vanishing. Three months later, I have no pain or swollen joints in my hands or feet, and I have no hot flashes in the day or night. It's wonderful.

I don't feel so anxious and my family notice that I am much calmer. My concentration has also returned and with it my confidence, which had all but gone. I feel that I've been given my old life back and am very grateful.

Problem	Supplement	Daily Dose
General symptoms of the menopause	Gynovite multivitamin & mineral supplement (US), Swiss One "10" Classic Multi (Canada)	2-4 per day 2 per day
Hot flashes & night sweats	Isoflavone-rich supplements, such as Promensil	1 per day which delivers 40mg of isoflavones
Hot flashes & night sweats	Sage Oil	1-2ml (28-56 drops) 2-3 times per day
Vaginal dryness	Omega-7	2 capsules twice per day
Vaginal dryness	Arkopharma Phyto Soya Vaginal Gel	Inserted twice per week
Menstrual disorders	Agnus Castus	54mg of fresh herb
Libido & depression	Hypericum (St John's Wort)	900mg per day
Aches & pains	Glucosamine Sulphate	400mg 3 times per day
Aches & pains	Cardiozen, strong fish oils	750mg twice per day
Loss of libido	Horny Goat Weed	600mg per day

Problem	Supplement	Daily Dose
Loss of libido	ArginMax	3 in morning & 3 at night
Osteoporosis	Promensil, Calcium & magnesium supplement	1 per day 1-2 per day
Dry skin	Arkopharma Phyto Soy Face Cream & body lotion	Apply daily
Insomnia	Valerian	600mg at night
Heavy periods	Magnesium, amino acid & chelate	2 x 150mg tablets per day
Heavy periods	Vitex Agnus Castus	1,000mg
Heavy periods	Iron-Ferrous Sulphate	1 x 200mg tablet with fruit juice
Constipation	Magnesium, amino acid, & chelate	2-6 x 150mg tablets at night

The supplements are available at our online shop www.askmaryonstewart.com/member or through our mail order company (see page 370 for details). If you are a member of Maryon Stewart's Lifebay you will receive discounts on all of our products.

"I had early menopause and developed a very dry vagina, to the point where intercourse made me bleed. It was so sore and painful that I was completely put off sex, which obviously put a strain on my relationship. Maryon suggested I try Arkopharma Vaginal Gel as part of my program. I noticed an improvement within the first month. Within three months, my vaginal tissues were back to normal. It's made an enormous difference and I'm delighted."

Kate Waters

Other Useful Herbs

A number of other herbs can alleviate symptoms of both perimenopause and menopause:

Licorice Root

Also known as Glycyrrhiza Glabra and sarsaparilla root, this contains phytoestrogen and can be used in conjunction with other herbs and brewed into herbal tea. However, licorice can cause sodium retention and increases the risk of high blood pressure in some people.

Dong Quai

Also known as Angelica Polymorphia, this contains phytoestrogen and is considered in Chinese medicine to be a harmonising tonic. It has traditionally been used to treat female complaints, such as heavy bleeding and PMS, and now has a place in the treatment of menopause symptoms.

Sage Leaf

Also known as Salvia Officianalis, this member of the mint family contains estrogenic substances that can help relieve hot flashes and night sweats. In a study carried out on the medicinal uses of plant drugs, 40 patients were given dried aqueous extract of fresh sage (440mg) and 40 were given infusion of sage (4.5g) daily. Both groups of patients experienced a reduction in sweating.

Vitex Agnus Castus

Research has found this can significantly relieve symptoms of PMS, such as irritability, mood swings, headaches, breast fullness, abdominal cramps and depression. Results are usually noticeable within three cycles, making it useful for perimenopause.

Valerian

This is a traditional herbal remedy for symptomatic relief of stress and tension, promoting natural sleep without the unpleasant side-effects of more conventional drugs. It can also be taken for anxiety and conditions worsened by stress, such as irritable bowel syndrome.

Panax Ginseng

This can be moderately helpful in controlling hot flashes, especially when used in conjunction with natural Vitamin E.

St John's Wort

Also known as Hypericum, this has been used in treating depression for many years. It is thought to be more effective in treating moderate depression and has fewer side-effects than conventional anti-depressants. A 12-week German study of 111 women experiencing libido problems at the time of menopause found that 60% of the women using St John's Wort significantly regained their libido.

Black Cohosh has been a promising herbal supplement for the reduction of menopausal symptoms. However, a US trial published in June 2006 came up blank. In this trial, the 132 women receiving Black Cohosh showed a 20% improvement over four weeks, slightly less than those receiving a placebo.

The UK medicines watchdog, the MHRA, stated in July 2006 that all products containing Black Cohosh should carry a warning. Two committees examined the safety data and confirmed that liver injury or failure is a rare, but a serious side-effect. If you display symptoms of liver injury, such as pain on the right side of your stomach, unexplained nausea, flu-symptoms, dark urine or yellowing of the eyes or skin, stop taking this remedy.

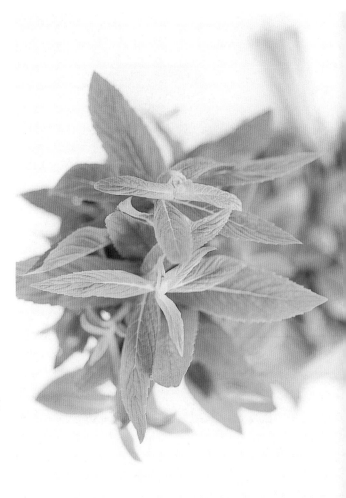

"After being woken by night sweats repeatedly in the beginning, it became very difficult for me to get back to sleep. Maryon suggested I take some Valerian in the night to help me relax enough to doze off again and I was relieved to find that it did work. I didn't need to continue in the long-term as I am no longer disturbed by hot sweats in the night and I am sleeping better now than I have for so long."

Betty Evans

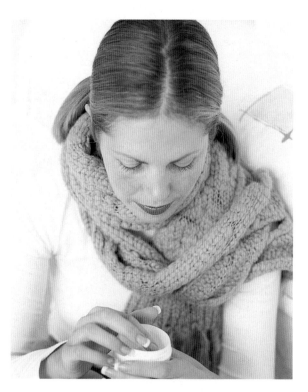

Wrinkle Rescue

By the time you reach menopause, you will have collected a number of wrinkles or 'wisdom stripes' as I prefer to call them. The cosmetic industry is very aware that most of us are eager to camouflage these and reverse the aging appearance of our skin as much as possible. As a result, there are many face and body creams on the market, varying in price from quite reasonable to incredibly expensive.

The cream I use and recommend is Arkopharma Age Minimizing Cream because clinical trials have found it reduces the depths of wrinkles by up to 48% within four weeks. It is very popular with women in our clinic as it feels good on the skin and it makes the skin feel smooth, soft and more youthful. The other reason we all like it is it only costs a fraction of the price of many other creams marketed by cosmetic houses.

Sarah Adams, York

During my menopause, I noticed that the condition of my skin began to deteriorate. Eventually, it became abrasive to the touch and had a red appearance. It felt very uncomfortable and made me feel self-conscious at a time when I was feeling far from my best because of my menopause

Maryon Stewart was helping me sort out my general symptoms and when I mentioned my skin problems (we had never met because my consultations were by telephone), she suggested I use Arkopharma Age Minimizing Cream. I initially used it once a day and it did help to some degree. Maryon then suggested I use it twice a day. Within a few weeks, I had an absolute success on my hands! People now comment on how great my skin looks, which has boosted my confidence and made me feel so much better.

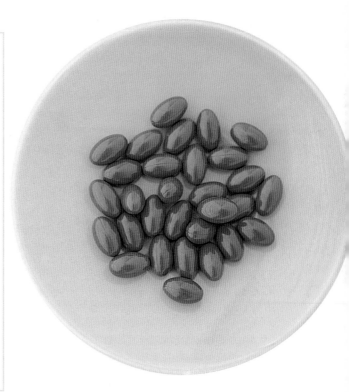

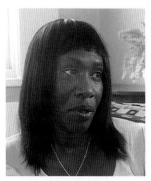

Marva's Story

About a year before she came to see me, Marva Morrison, 48, had a radical hysterectomy (due to fibroids and heavy bleeding) and a hormone implant as a consequence of this.

After the hysterectomy, I felt like a different person in every way. I got very depressed and wished I hadn't agreed to have my ovaries removed. They said I should have them removed as I might get cancer, so I went along with it, but they were healthy ovaries and I really regretted it.

I had so many symptoms - I was anxious and irritable, I had frequent headaches, I couldn't sleep, which was made worse by the fact that I had to go to the bathroom at least twice during the night. I also experienced hot flashes when the implant wore off. My vagina was constantly itchy, I wasn't interested in sex and I had thrush fairly regularly. My memory was awful, I couldn't concentrate and my confidence was really low. I lost my job before the operation, which made me feel even worse.

After my first consultation with Maryon, I stopped eating wheat for a while and ate more fresh food and oily fish. I added flaxseeds and soy products to my diet during the day and started doing regular exercise and a session of relaxation each day.

Fairly soon after I began the program, I started feeling much better, but I had the flu shortly after, then hurt my back. However, I kept on going and I visited a cranial osteopath, who helped with my headaches and my back. I soon noticed how much energy I had, I stopped flashing and I no longer needed to go to the bathroom during the night. I felt less stressed and much more like my normal self. I now look after two of my young grandchildren full-time and am amazed that I can cope, since I never would have been able to before.

The supplements really helped. For example, I noticed a big improvement when I took the Promensil, as the flashes calmed down and I was able to sleep through the night. My vagina stopped itching and the thrush cleared up. The fish oils helped with my joints and mobility, and the St John's Wort and the exercise seemed to ease my depression. The whole program made a huge difference to my life and I'm very grateful.

"I went into an early menopause, which brought with it many unpleasant symptoms, including vaginal dryness and loss of libido. Sexual intercourse became very painful and uncomfortable, which put a strain on my marriage, especially as my husband is five years younger than I am. Even within the first month of taking Omega-7, I noticed a significant improvement. My vagina was no longer dry and sex became more comfortable and therefore much more regular again."

Jean Krane

"Every woman needs to give herself time
to make the transition into midlife."

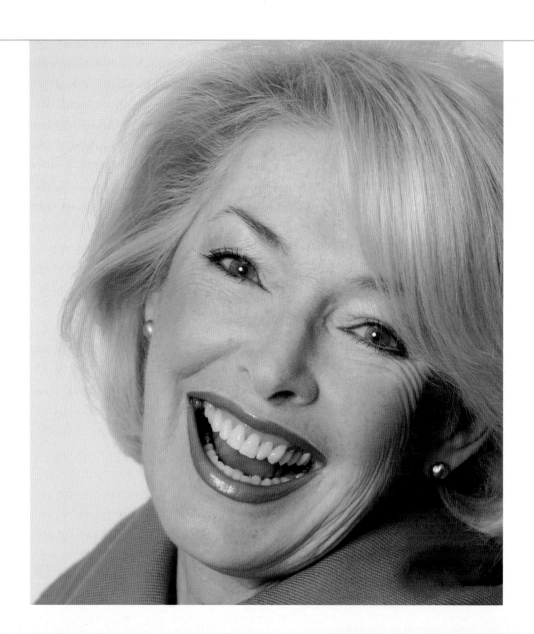

frequently asked questions

Q. How long does it have to be after my last period before I know I've been through menopause? I keep thinking my periods have finished, but I seem to have a period every four or five months.

A. The general consensus is that you should consider you have passed your menopause when you have stopped menstruating for one year. Menopause is actually the last day of your last period, so it can only be dated in hindsight.

Q. I've been taking HRT for the last five years and would like to stop, but I'm not sure whether to stop suddenly or come off gradually.

A. It is wise to wean yourself gradually off HRT, since research shows that coming off HRT suddenly is likely to worsen hot flashes. At the NHAS, we usually establish patients on a phytoestrogen-rich program for the first month. This includes taking recommended supplements and undertaking a daily session of formal relaxation, and then reducing your HRT dose by half in the second month, before phasing it out altogether in the third month. Our most recent survey showed we were able to wean over 91% of women off HRT seamlessly within five months.

Q. I take HRT, but I've also read about the importance of including phytoestrogen in my diet. Is it wise to do both or should I just do one or the other?

A. As far as I am aware, no research has ever been conducted to demonstrate that the two types of treatment conflict in any way. If you intend to stay on HRT and consume substantial amounts of phytoestrogen, you should ask your doctor about possibly adjusting the dose of your HRT.

Q. How much phytoestrogen do I need each day to control my hot flashes?

A. The dose of isoflavone in trials varies from 30mg to 170mg per day. It takes about 100mg of isoflavones per day to control severe hot flashes. This should be consumed through both food and supplements. Research confirms it is best to consume these in small quantities throughout the day, rather than in one sitting. A regular intake of isoflavones helps keep the blood estrogen levels elevated. As a rough guide, there are approximately 20mg of isoflavones in a 250ml glass of soy milk, 10mg in a small tub of soy yogurt or dessert, 25mg in 100gm of tofu and 7mg in a tablespoon of organic Golden Flaxseeds.

A. If your hot flashes, night sweats and vaginal dryness are controlled adequately by HRT, then you are receiving an effective dose. Symptoms such as breast tenderness, fluid retention and mood swings may indicate that your dose is too high and your doctor may wish to reduce the strength of your medication. Younger women typically require higher doses of HRT to control their symptoms. Occasionally, blood tests may be necessary to determine dosage adjustment.

A. HRT does help protect against bone loss in the short-term and it is thought to help improve bone mass by 3% while you're taking it. However, within five years of stopping HRT, your bones will return to how they would have been without the HRT. It used to be thought that HRT protected against heart disease, but recent research has found this is not the case and that in fact it can increase the risk of heart disease and stroke.

Incorporating phytoestrogen, which are naturally occurring, estrogen-like substances, into your daily diet has been shown in a number of preliminary studies to protect bones. A significant number of trials show this can also protect against heart disease and it also seems to protect against memory loss. In addition, Promensil supplements have been shown to help regenerate bone in the spine. Therefore, not taking HRT will not put you at further risk.

A. In theory, it is possible to overdose on many things, including water. However, if you stay within the range of phytoestrogen that has been tested in clinical trials, you should not suffer any adverse effects. Japanese adults consume an average of 10-20gm of soy protein per day. There are about 8gm of soy protein in a cup of soy milk and 10-12gm in a serving of tofu. We recommend 2 or 3 servings per day at regular intervals to meet the needs of the estrogen receptor sites.

A. Some, but not all, menopause supplements are standardised, which means they are prepared to pharmaceutical standards and have undergone clinical trials. We only recommend the most scientifically based supplements for our Natural Menopause Programme. We recommend Promensil, which provides 40mg of isoflavones and has undergone many trials around the world. Fot those who require more isoflavones, but cannot tolerate soy, or who often travel away from home, we also use Arkopharma's Phyto Soya capsules. These deliver either 17.5mg or 35mg per capsule and have also been through some positive clinical trials. Another option is Sage Leaf, which has also been shown to reduce hot flashes in clinical trials. These supplements can be taken in conjunction with each other at different times of the day. We tend not to use Black Cohosh as studies have found it may cause liver damage. It is certainly unsuitable for women who have a family history of breast cancer.

Q. Does everyone absorb isoflavones well or is there something I can do to improve their absorption in my body?

A. It seems that some people absorb isoflavones better than others. There are indeed ways of improving absorption. Alcohol and cigarettes both tend to impede absorption of estrogen and it has been well documented that a course of antibiotics can also disturb absorption for several months. Reducing alcohol consumption to only small quantities, minimizing or quitting smoking, and taking a supplement of probiotics after a course of antibiotics will help improve absorption.

Q. Can isoflavones be absorbed through your skin? If so, is this a way of protecting myself against menopausal symptoms?

A. Research is beginning to show that estrogen deficiencies in the skin can be corrected by applying specific phytoestrogen-rich creams, such as Arkopharma Age Minimizing Cream. It seems these creams increase production of new collagen cells and new skin cells, resulting in a significant reduction in wrinkles. Although this is good news, skin creams do not replace HRT or the need to consume a phytoestrogen-rich diet to control the unpleasant symptoms of menopause.

Q. I tried coming off HRT a couple of years ago, but developed a very dry vagina and sex became quite painful. I'm afraid this will happen again if I stop taking HRT. Is there anything else I can do to avoid this symptom?

A. Research published in 1990 in the British Medical Journal reported that a group of women taking soy products, linseeds and Promensil were able to bring about the same changes in their vaginal lining as women taking HRT. We incorporate all these products in our program with good effect. We also recommend Arkopharma's Phyto Soya Vaginal Gel, which is inserted in the vagina twice a week and has been shown to restore the lining of the vagina.

We also recommend a Scandinavian product made by PharmaNord called Omega-7, an extract from the marine Sea Buckthorn, which is taken daily in capsule form and encourages cells to produce mucous again. Making the necessary dietary changes and taking the recommended supplements is normally very satisfactory, but it takes a month or two to see a difference.

Q. I've been treated for breast cancer in the past, so should I be concerned about consuming phytoestrogen?

A. Genistein and daidzein, two key isoflavones found in soy products, are thought to block the uptake of estrogen in a similar way to the drug Tamoxifen, which is often administered to breast cancer sufferers. Research has shown these prevent the growth of cancer cells by inhibiting the activity of oncogenes, the genes that promote cancer, and other cancer-causing enzymes. Asian diets rich in isoflavones seem to have protective qualities. Far fewer women die of breast cancer in Korea, for example, than Western countries. But it is advisable to check with your doctor.

Q. I have thyroid problems and have heard that soy is likely to have an adverse effect. Is this true?

A. There has been a significant amount of research on thyroid function and soy. It seems that soy does not adversely affect thyroid function, but it may interfere with the action of synthetic thyroid hormones, just as fiber supplements or cholesterol-lowering drugs would. As a result, dosage of thyroid medication may need increasing by about 25%. This shouldn't present a problem, as medication dosage is determined by blood thyroid levels of each individual. There is no justified reason for someone with thyroid problems to avoid soy.

Q. Soy products seem to be one of the richest sources of isoflavones, but I'm wondering if I should be worried about recent concerns regarding genetically modified soy?

A. Some people prefer non-genetically modified soy for nutritional reasons, but we are not aware of any difference between GM and non-GM soy. It is likely that much of the recent research has involved GM soy and varying degrees of benefits have still been observed. Both varieties are now widely available and clearly labelled, so it is best for consumers to make their own choice based on preference until there is further evidence to guide expert recommendations.

Q. Soy products make my tummy bloated and gassy. Is there anything else I can use to get naturally occurring estrogen in my diet?

A. Soy can initially cause this reaction, but symptoms usually calm down within a few weeks. You could try heating the soy milk and adding some ginger, which is often more tolerable, or try flaxseeds, a rich source of naturally occurring estrogen. A tablespoon of flaxseeds with your breakfast cereal and another in the afternoon with some yogurt or on a salad will go a long way to providing your daily requirements, in conjunction with taking a Promensil pill each day, which provides another 40mg of isoflavones.

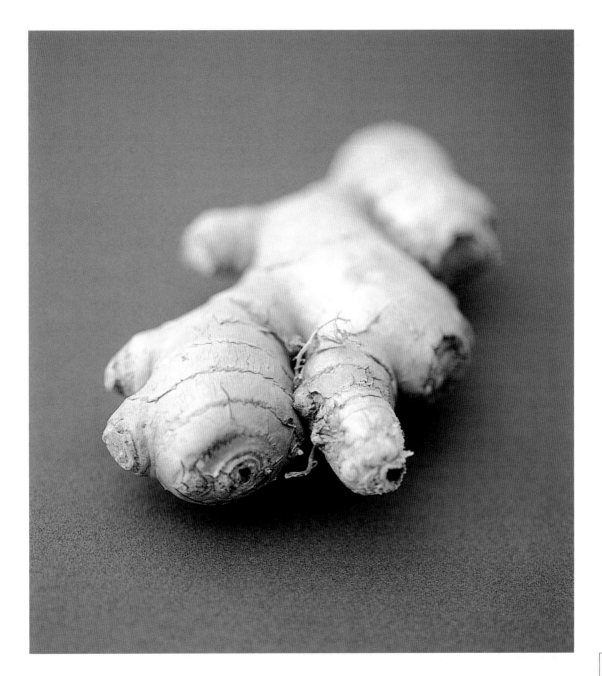

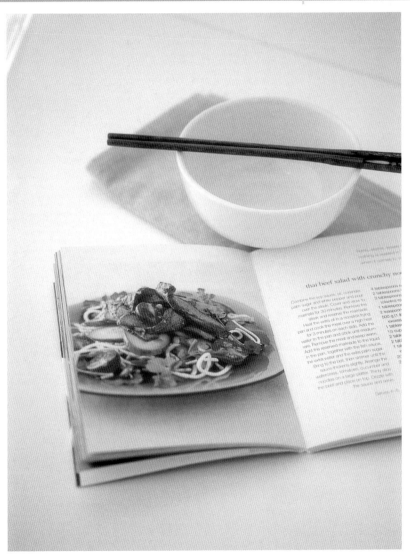

"Over and Over – feeling alive

Over and Over – courage survives

Over and Over – change of the heart

Over and Over – here I start

Here in my heart

Sue Fisher Hendry

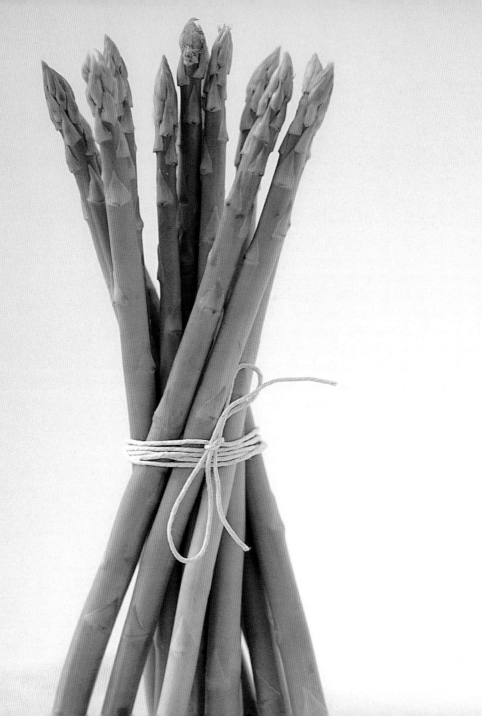

phyto-rich menu plans

Plants such as soy, flaxseeds and red clover, are collectively known as phytoestrogen rich as they contain naturally occurring estrogens known as isoflavones and lignans. Foods rich in these important naturally occurring estrogen-like substances have been found to significantly reduce menopausal symptoms for many who include them into their diet.

You don't need to radically change your diet to increase your intake, just make a few modifications here and there. Start by becoming familiar with the phyto-rich foods that you most enjoy eating, a large variety of which are readily available in supermarkets, then look at how you can most easily include these in your diet.

Following are some recommended meal plans to help you incorporate more isoflavones and lignans into your daily menu. There are a number of simple but delicious recipes for you to try, which all contain naturally occurring estrogen.

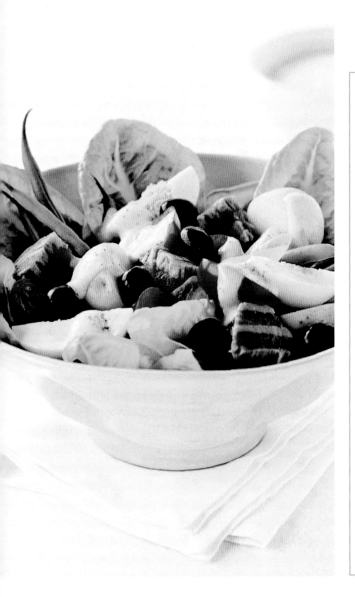

Lunches

Fast Options

- Raw vegetables and dips eg. hummus, taramasalata
- Refried soy beans with corn tacos
- Jacket potato with spicy soy beans
- Jacket potato with barbecue soy beans
- Omelette with salad (see salad selection)
- Spicy soy beans on rye toast
- Stir-fry tofu and mixed vegetables with rice
- Soup and rye, corn or soy bread
- Rice salad with pumpkin seeds, sunflower seeds and nuts
- Fruit and nut compote with soy yogurt
- Scrambled tofu with rye bread or jacket potato
- Soy and buckwheat pancakes with refried soy beans
- Grilled tempeh with salad
- Bean tacos with salad
- Tempeh kebab with pitta bread
- Sesame tofu with salad
- Rye bread with soy cheese and salad
- Oatcakes with nut butter and salad

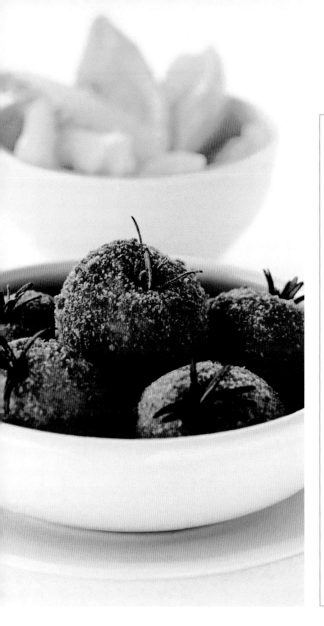

Dinners

Fast Options

- Tofu kebabs with satay sauce and stir-fried vegetables and rice
- Tofu risotto
- Shrimp and tofu kebabs with rice and salad
- Lamb kebabs with vegetables and rice
- Salmon steaks with orange ginger sauce and vegetables
- Refried beans with rice, corn fries and avocado
- Stir-fried tofu and vegetables with rice noodles
- Tofu burgers with salad and a jacket potato
- Baked avocado with tuna, salad and a jacket potato
- Stuffed bell pepper with salad
- Grilled lamb chop with rosemary, vegetables and new potatoes
- Chicken kebabs with tamari and ginger dressing
- Spinach gratin with a jacket potato
- Tofu, bean and herb stir-fry with rice
- Noodles in spicy sesame sauce
- Cauliflower cheese with a jacket potato
- Sesame tofu with salad and a jacket potato

Week 1

Day 1

Breakfast
Oatmeal made with soy milk
Almonds
Sunflower seeds, pumpkin seeds
Banana, chopped

Lunch
Cauliflower soup*
Oatcakes or French bread
Apple

Dinner
Chicken with almond sauce
Green beans
Sweetcorn
Jacket potato

Dessert
Cinnamon rhubarb with soy yogurt

Snacks
Dried apricots
Almond biscuit

Day 2

Breakfast
Soy yogurt
Apple, chopped
Sunflower seeds, pumpkin seeds
Pecan nuts, chopped

Lunch
Scrambled tofu
Pilchards

Dinner
Polenta pie
Rice
Roasted vegetables

Dessert
Prune and tofu dessert*

Snacks
Orange
Honey soy loaf
Revival Soy Shake

Day 3

Breakfast
Crunchy almond muesli* with soy milk
Pear, chopped

Lunch
Jacket potato
Refried soy beans
Green salad
Apple

Dinner
Baked chicken burgers with almond chili dressing
Rice
Sweetcorn
Broccoli

Dessert
Apple and cinnamon crumble with soy custard

Snacks
Pear
Rice cakes with nut butter
Sunflower seeds, pumpkin seeds

* Recipes are in the recipe section (chapter 24)

Day 4

Breakfast
Banana oat pancakes* with soy yogurt and chopped fresh fruit

Lunch
Sesame tofu with tahini mayonnaise
Tropical rice salad*
Apple

Dinner
Soy bean casserole
New potatoes
Peas
Carrots

Dessert
Blackberry and rhubarb compote
Soy Dream or soy yogurt

Snacks
Banana
Mixed unsalted nuts
Revival Soy Crispy Bar

Day 5

Breakfast
Rice porridge made with soy milk
Dried apricots
Almonds
Sesame seeds

Lunch
Watercress soup*
Soy and cornbread
Small piece of cheese
Apple

Dinner
Baked avocado with tuna
Endive, fruit and nut salad
New potatoes

Dessert
Tofu orange almond dessert

Snacks
Oatcakes with pure fruit spread
Banana

Day 6

Breakfast
Soy and raisin loaf
Banana smoothie with phyto sprinkle*

Lunch
Jacket potato with spicy soy beans*
Coleslaw

Dinner
Shepherdess pie
Cauliflower
Carrots

Dessert
Banana and tofu cream

Snacks
Sesame squares
Revival Soy Shake
Revival Soy Crispy Bar

Day 7

Breakfast
Crunchy almond muesli* with soy milk
Pear, chopped

Lunch
Burgen bread
Soy cheese
Apple and nut salad*

Dinner
Salmon potato cakes with avocado sauce
Tropical rice salad

Dessert
Ginger fruit salad
Soy Dream

Snacks
Cinnamon flapjack
Banana and date shake

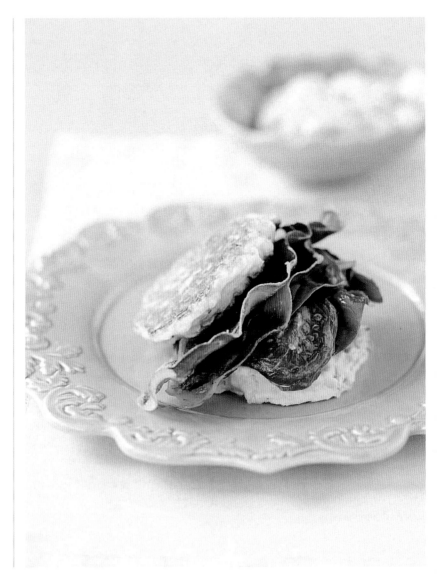

* Recipes are in the recipe section (chapter 24)

Week 2

Day 1

Breakfast
Phyto Muesli* with soy milk
Pear, chopped

Lunch
Tempeh kebab with pitta bread
Apple

Dinner
Shrimp and almond risotto
Green beans
Sweetcorn

Dessert
Banana and rice pudding*

Snacks
Buckwheat soy scone with
pure fruit jam
Pear

Day 2

Breakfast
Cornflakes with soy milk
Raisins
Pecan nuts
Sunflower seeds, pumpkin
seeds

Lunch
Bean tacos with green salad
Apple

Dinner
Salmon steaks with orange and
ginger sauce
New potatoes
Zucchini
Carrots

Dessert
Fruit and nut compote
Soy yogurt

Snacks
Dried apricots
Chocolate fruit slice
Revival Soy Crispy Bar

Day 3

Breakfast
Puffed rice cereal with soy milk
Banana, chopped
Pecan nuts, chopped
Phyto sprinkle*

Lunch
Herbed tofu pâté
Oatcakes
Rice salad with pumpkin seeds,
sunflower seeds and nuts

Dinner
Yogurt roast chicken
Swede
Roast potatoes
Carrots
Cabbage

Dessert
Rhubarb fool with tofu lemon
sauce

Snacks
Ginger snaps
Apple

Day 4

Breakfast
Oatmeal made with soy milk
Almonds
Dried apricots
Phyto sprinkle

Lunch
Scrambled tofu
Oatcakes and soy cheese
Apple

Dinner
Lamb stir-fry with almonds and walnuts
Rice noodles

Dessert
Tofu strawberry dessert

Snacks
Barley scone with pure fruit spread
Banana

Day 5

Breakfast
Cornflakes with soy milk
Banana, chopped
Almonds
Phyto sprinkle*

Lunch
Jacket potato with barbecue soy beans*
Green salad
Apple

Dinner
Nutty tofu risotto
Orange and avocado salad*

Dessert
Banana lemon whip

Snacks
Chewy fruit bar*
Pear
Revival Soy Crispy Bar

Day 6

Breakfast
Scrambled tofu
Grilled tomato and mushrooms
Grilled tempeh
Slice of toast

Lunch
Carrot soup
Soy and cornbread
Soy cheese

Dinner
Shrimp and spinach curry
Rice
Poppadam

Dessert
Apricot squares with soy custard

Snacks
Honey loaf, toasted
Mixed nuts

* Recipes are in the recipe section (chapter 24)

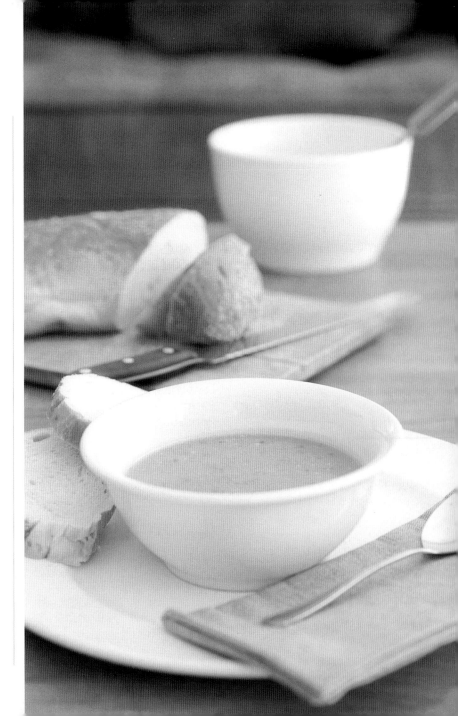

Day 7

Breakfast
Soy yogurt
Fresh fruit of your choice
Almonds and pecan nuts
Phyto sprinkle*

Lunch
Hummus* and raw vegetables
Oatcakes
Apple

Dinner
Stuffed bell pepper
Rice
Green beans
Sweetcorn

Dessert
Apple and tofu cheesecake

Snacks
Apricot coconut balls
Banana
Revival Soy Shake

Week 3

Day 1

Breakfast
Rice porridge made with
soy milk
Dried apricots
Almonds, chopped

Lunch
Soy and buckwheat pancakes
with refried soy beans
Green salad
Pear

Dinner
Lamb kebabs with
mint yogurt sauce
Rice
Sweetcorn
Green beans

Dessert
Rhubarb and ginger mousse

Snacks
Fruit smoothie
Oatcakes with nut butter

Day 2

Breakfast
Phyto Muesli* with soy milk
Banana, chopped

Lunch
Jacket potato with spicy soy
beans*
Endive, fruit and nut salad

Dinner
Lentil dhal
Basmati rice
Poppadam

Dessert
Chocolate pie with
passionfruit sauce

Snacks
Seed bread, toasted with pure
fruit spread
Dried apricots
Revival Soy Crispy Bar

Day 3

Breakfast
Cornflakes with soy milk
Banana, chopped
Almonds
Phyto sprinkle*

Lunch
Tofu tuna spread
Rye bread
Green salad

Dinner
Grilled tuna steak with orange
sauce
New potatoes
Carrots
Broccoli

Dessert
Ginger fruit salad
Soy Dream or soy yogurt

Snacks
Rice, soy and raisin bread with
pure fruit spread
Apple
Sunflower seeds and
pumpkin seeds

* Recipes are in the recipe section (chapter 24)

Day 4

Breakfast
Soy yogurt
Apple
Almonds
Apple bread roll*

Lunch
Herbed tofu pâté with crudités
Rye bread, toasted
Pear

Dinner
Lasagne
Green salad

Dessert
Créme caramel

Snacks
Almond biscuit
Banana
Revival Soy Shake

Day 5

Breakfast
Scrambled tofu
Grilled mushrooms
Rye bread, toasted

Lunch
Potato skins with broccoli and
tofu filling
Green salad
Apple

Dinner
Italian corn pasta
Sweetcorn
Broccoli

Dessert
Rhubarb crumble
Soy Dream or soy custard

Snacks
Banana smoothie
Barley scone

Day 6

Breakfast
Crunchy almond muesli* with
soy yogurt
Banana, chopped

Lunch
Lentil soup
Rye bread, toasted
Apple and nut salad

Dinner
Spicy chili*
Green salad
Sweetcorn

Dessert
Elderflower sorbet*
Soy Dream

Snacks
Rhubarb and blueberry
smoothie*
Apple

Day 7

Banana oat pancakes* with
soy yogurt and honey

Leek, sweetcorn and almond
soup
Rye bread toasted
Pear

Lentil bolognese
Green salad

Apricot squares
Soy custard

Honey loaf
Apple
Revival Soy Shake

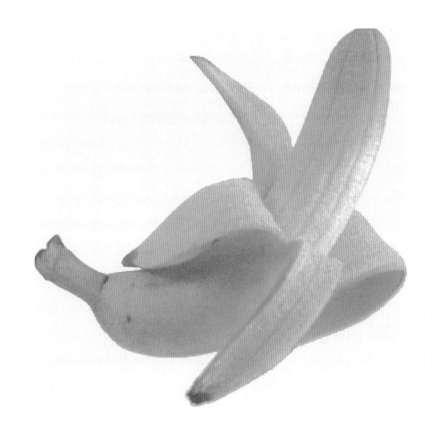

* Recipes are in the recipe section (chapter 24)

Day 1

Breakfast
Cornflakes with soy milk
Dried apricots
Almonds

Lunch
Soy bean and vegetable soup
Rye bread
Apple

Dinner
Shrimp and tofu kebabs with
peanut chili sauce
Rice
Sweetcorn
Green salad

Dessert
Banana and tofu cream

Snacks
Ginger snaps
Mixed nuts
Revival Soy Crispy Bar

Day 2

Breakfast
Puffed rice cereal with soy milk
Banana, chopped
Pecans, chopped

Lunch
Sesame tofu with salad
Pear

Dinner
Lamb stir-fry with almonds and
walnuts
Rice
Zucchini
Carrots

Dessert
Fruit and nut compote
Soy Dream or soy yogurt

Snacks
Honey loaf
Pear

Day 3

Breakfast
Phyto Muesli* with soy milk
Banana, chopped

Lunch
Hummus* with crudités
Oatcakes
Apple

Dinner
Chicken kebabs with tamari
and ginger dressing
Jacket potato
Brown rice and watercress
salad*

Dessert
Banana and rice pudding*
Dried apricots, chopped

Snacks
Apple
Mixed unsalted nuts
Revival Soy Crispy Bar

Day 4

Breakfast
Breakfast rice cakes with soy yogurt and pure fruit spread
Banana

Lunch
Carrot and apricot pâté
Oatcakes
Green salad

Dinner
Lamb steaks with pomegranate and walnut sauce
Green beans
Broccoli
Carrots

Dessert
Apple and tofu cheesecake
Soy Dream

Snacks
Buckwheat scone
Soy yogurt with chopped dried apricots and mixed nuts

Day 5

Breakfast
Oatmeal made with soy milk
Dried apricots
Almonds

Lunch
Jacket potato with barbecue soy beans*
Green salad
Banana

Dinner
Chicken and almond pilaff
Sweetcorn
Green beans

Dessert
Chocolate and fruit slice

Snacks
Honey loaf, toasted
Apple

Day 6

Breakfast
Phyto Muesli* with soy milk
Banana, chopped

Lunch
Watercress soup*
Seed bread*, toasted

Dinner
Tuna and lentil bake
Jacket potato
Broccoli

Dessert
Ginger fruit salad with Soy Dream

Snacks
Almond loaf
Banana
Revival Soy Shake

* Recipes are in the recipe section (chapter 24)

Day 7

Breakfast
Soy yogurt
Kiwi fruit, banana, chopped
Almonds, pumpkin seeds
Dried apricots

Lunch
Rye bread sandwich with
tofu tuna spread
Apple and nut salad

Dinner
Soy bean biryani
Vegetable curry
Poppadam

Dessert
Prune and tofu dessert*

Snacks
Sesame square
Pear

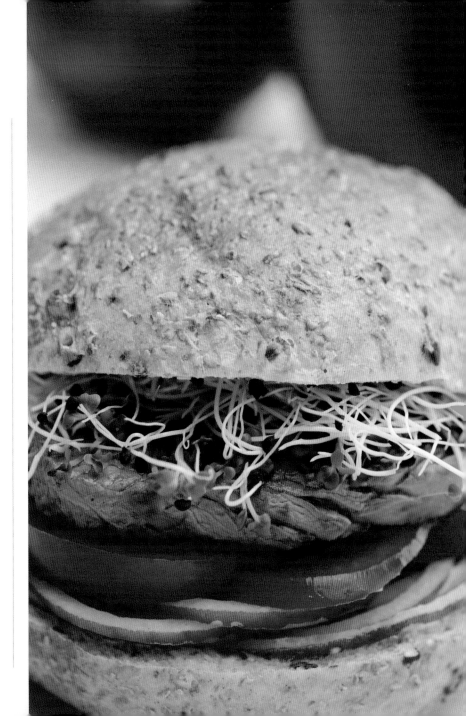

Vegetarian Sample Menu - 2 Weeks

Week 1

Day 1

Breakfast
Scrambled tofu
Grilled tomatoes and
mushrooms
Rye bread, toasted

Lunch
Hummus* with crudités
Oatcakes
Apple

Dinner
Tofu, bean and herb stir-fry
Rice

Dessert
Rhubarb and ginger whip
Soy Dream

Snacks
Apricot and coconut balls
Pear
Revival Soy Crispy Bar

Day 2

Breakfast
Rice porridge with soy milk
Raisins, dried apricots

Lunch
Chick pea soup
Soy and cornbread
Soy cheese

Dinner
Spinach gratin
Jacket potato
Carrots
Sweetcorn

Dessert
Stewed apple and blackberries
with soy custard

Snacks
Apple bread roll* with pure
fruit spread
Almonds

Day 3

Breakfast
Dried fruit compote
Almonds
Soy yogurt

Lunch
Savoury crackers
Soy cheese
Orange and avocado salad*

Dinner
Hungarian bean goulash
Saute potatoes
Cauliflower
Carrots

Dessert
Rhubarb fool with
tofu lemon cream

Snacks
Almond and cinnamon flapjack
Banana

* Recipes are in the recipe section (chapter 24)

Day 4

Breakfast
Cornflakes and puffed
rice cereal with
soy milk
Almonds, pecan nuts
Dried apricots

Lunch
Carrot and almond pâté
Oatcakes
Green salad

Dinner
Leek gratin
New potatoes
Carrots
Zucchini

Dessert
Chocolate tofu berry whip

Snacks
Sesame slice
Apple

Day 5

Breakfast
Poached egg
Rye bread, toasted
Banana

Lunch
Brown rice and watercress salad
½ avocado
Apple bread roll*

Dinner
Carrot and nut loaf with
tahini and lemon dressing
Sweet potato salad
Zucchini

Dessert
Tofu cheesecake
Soy Dream

Snacks
Soy yogurt
Dried apricots
Almonds

Day 6

Breakfast
Soy yogurt
Banana and pear, chopped
Oatcakes and marmalade

Lunch
Jacket potato
Mackerel in tomato sauce
Apple, carrot and ginger salad

Dinner
Barley roast with tahini sauce
New potatoes
Sweetcorn
Broccoli

Dessert
Nut crunch with
tofu whipped cream

Snacks
Almond biscuit
Pear
Mixed nuts

Day 7

Phyto Muesli* with soy milk
Pear, chopped

Jacket potato with hummus*
Green salad
Apple

Indonesian tofu kebabs with
satay sauce
Stir-fried mixed vegetables
Rice noodles

Rhubarb crumble
with soy custard

Fruit chewy bar*
Pear
Revival Soy Shake

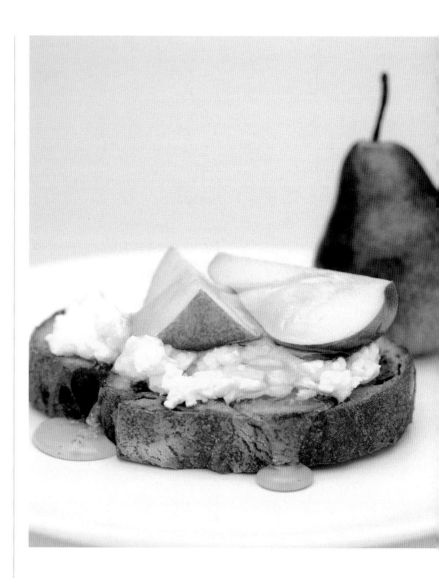

* Recipes are in the recipe section (chapter 24)

Day 1

Breakfast
Rice porridge with soy milk
Banana, chopped
Almonds

Lunch
Leek, sweetcorn and
almond soup
Rye bread, toasted
Apple

Dinner
Broccoli and smoked tofu
New potatoes
Carrots
Sweetcorn

Dessert
Brown rice pudding

Snacks
Apricot and coconut balls
Pear

Day 2

Breakfast
Oatmeal made with soy milk
Banana, chopped
Dried apricots

Lunch
Jacket potato
Tuna in soy oil
Green salad
Apple

Dinner
Shepherdess pie
Carrots
Cabbage

Dessert
Tofu-orange and almond
dessert*

Snacks
Sesame squares
Pear

Day 3

Breakfast
Cornflakes with soy milk
Almonds
Banana, chopped

Lunch
Fennel, leek and celery soup
Soy and cornbread
Apple

Dinner
Noodles in spicy sesame sauce
Stir-fried mixed vegetables

Dessert
Oatmeal pudding

Snacks
Honey loaf
Pear

Day 4

Breakfast
Banana oat pancakes*
with soy yogurt
Apple

Lunch
Carrot and apricot pate
Rye bread, toasted
Pear

Dinner
Red lentil dhal with
basmati rice
Poppadam

Dessert
Banana raisin whip

Snacks
Oatcakes with pure fruit spread
Dried apricots
Mixed unsalted nuts

Day 5

Breakfast
Cornflakes with soy milk
Dried apricots
Pumpkin seeds and pecan nuts

Lunch
Scrambled tofu*
Rye bread, toasted
Endive, fruit and nut salad
Apple

Dinner
Lentil bolognaise
Spaghetti

Dessert
Cinnamon rhubarb whip

Snacks
Chocolate fruit slice
Pear

Day 6

Breakfast
Breakfast rice cakes with
mashed banana
Nut butter

Lunch
Jacket potato with hummus*
Orange and avocado salad*

Dinner
Zucchini and tomato quiche
Jacket potato
Endive, fruit and nut salad

Dessert
Raspberry and tofu brulée

Snacks
Orange and ginger cake
Apple

* Recipes are in the recipe section (chapter 24)

Day 7

Rice porridge
Banana, chopped
Almonds

Tropical rice salad
Sardines
Apple

Bean and tofu casserole
Jacket potato
Green beans
Carrots

Prune and tofu dessert*

Nutty flapjack
Banana

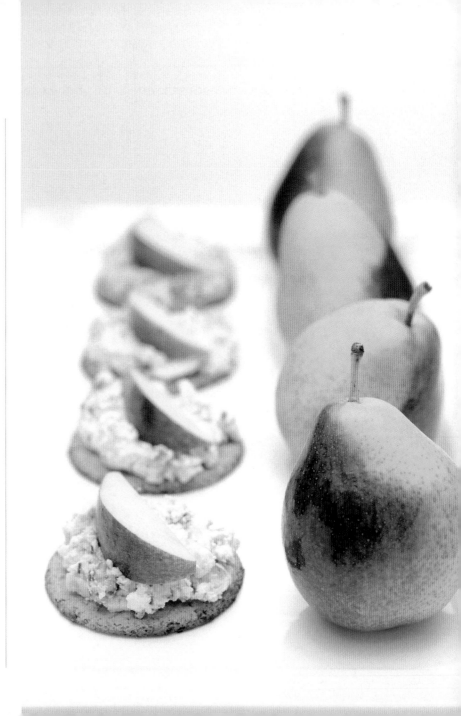

Putting Isoflavones on the Menu

The following three example menus outline the extent that phytoestrogen content can vary between menus.

Soy-Rich Vegetarian Menu

Qty		SF	TF	Protein	Carb	Fibre	Phyto
	Breakfast						
2oz (¼cup)	Oatmeal	0.1	2.5	7	27	2.3	Trace
150ml (¼pt)	Soy milk	0.25	2.3	3.3	2	1.3	10mg
1oz (⅛cup)	Almonds*	0.7	5.1	3.4	12	1.7	*
1 medium	Apple*	0.1	0.5	0.3	21	1.06	*
	Lunch						
3oz (⅓cup)	Hummus	1.1	4.1	14	9	1.75	15mg
1 slice	Rye bread	0	0.9	2.1	11	1.6	1mg
4oz (½cup)	Carrot and raisin salad	0.5	7.5	2.75	10.5	1.25	
	Dinner						
4oz	Indonesian tofu kebabs with satay sauce	5	14	27.2	17.3	1.2	50mg
4oz (½cup)	Stir-fried mixed vegetables	1.6	3.6	3.9	19.5	3	
4oz (½cup)	Basmati rice	0.1	0.4	4.8	45	0.21	Trace
	Dessert						
4oz (½cup)	Soy yogurt	0.6	3.6	5	3.9	0	12mg
	Snacks						
1 medium	Banana	0.2	0.6	1.2	27	0.57	
Kcal		92	405	300	829		

Total calories   1,626

Expressed as a percentage of total calories

Total Fat (TF)   23%

Saturated Fat (SF)   5%

Protein   18%

Carbohydrates   51%

Phytoestrogen (mg/day)   93mg

*contain phytoestrogen, but no published figures, so an additional 5mg per day is allowed

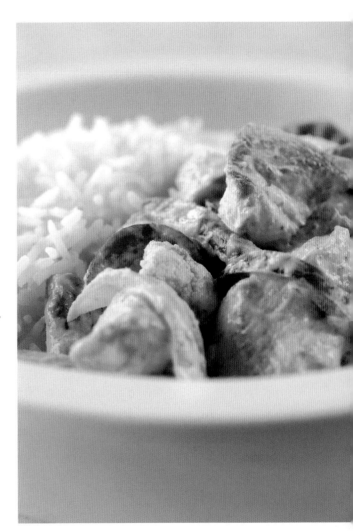

Soy-Rich Non-vegetarian Menu

Qty		SF	TF	Protein	Carb	Fibre	Phyto
	Breakfast						
2oz (¼cup)	Oatmeal	0.1	2.5	7	27	2.3	Trace
150ml (¼ pt)	Soy milk	0.25	2.3	3.3	2	1.3	10mg
1oz (⅛cup)	Almonds*	0.7	5.1	3.4	12	1.7	
1 medium	Pear	0	0	0.7	25	2.3	
	Lunch						
2 slices	Wholemeal bread	0	2.0	6	28	3.2	Trace
2oz (¼cup)	Cheddar cheese	12	16.4	14	0	0	
4oz (½cup)	Green salad	0	0	0.1	1	0.5	
1 medium	Apple*	0.1	0.5	0.3	21	1.06	
	Dinner						
4oz (½cup)	Chicken and tofu burger	6.5	12.1	27.2	3.5	0.6	11mg
1 medium	Jacket potato	0.1	0.2	4.7	51	1.2	
3oz (⅓cup)	Green beans	0.1	0.2	1.2	5	1.1	
3oz (⅓cup)	Sweetcorn	0.2	1.1	2.7	21	0.5	
	Dessert						
1 large	Stewed apple	0.5	0.1	0.5	51	1.2	
75ml (3fl oz)	Soy Dream*	0.75	8	1.5	1	0	13mg
	Snacks						
4oz (½cup)	Soy yogurt	0.6	3.6	5	3.9	0	12mg
1	Bagel	0	2.6	11	56	0.22	
Kcal		207	510	351	1,218		

Total calories   2,286

Expressed as a percentage of total calories

Total Fat (TF)   22%

Saturated Fat (SF)   9%

Protein   15%

Carbohydrates   53%

Phytoestrogen (mg/day)   51mg

*contain phytoestrogen, but no published figures,
so an additional 5mg per day is allowed

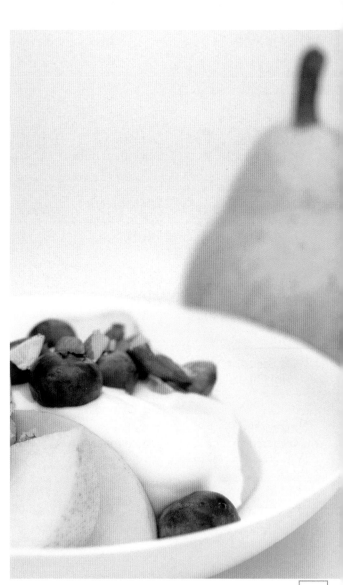

Typical Western Menu - Using Home Cooked Ingredients

Qty		SF	TF	Protein	Carbo	Fibre	Phyto
	Breakfast						
2oz (¼cup)	Oatmeal	0.1	2.5	7	27	2.3	Trace
150ml (¼ pt)	Full cream milk	2.5	4.1	4	5.5	0	
	Lunch						
2 slices	White bread	0	0.18	4	24	0.15	Trace
2 slices	Bacon	1.3	4	11.7	0	0	
1	Fried egg	2.4	6.4	5.4	0	0	
	Dinner						
4oz (½cup)	Steak	8.4	17	22	0	0	
4oz (½cup)	Fries	7	13	2.6	24	0	
3oz (⅓cup)	Peas	0	0	4.1	11	1.7	
	Dessert						
4oz (½cup)	Apple pie	4.7	17	3.4	61	0.6	
75ml (3fl oz)	Double cream	12	2.5	6	7	0	
	Snacks						
1 standard	Mars Bar	7.6	11	5	17	0	
4oz (½cup)	Whole milk yogurt	1.7	2.5	6	7	0	
Kcal		429	727	324	708		

Total calories   2,188

Expressed as a percentage of total calories

Total fat (TF)   33%

Saturated fat (SF)   19%

Protein   15%

Carbohydrates   32%

Phytoestrogen mg/day   Trace

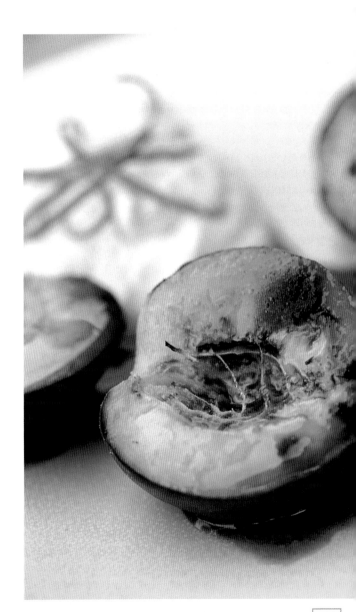

Breakfast

Phyto Muesli with a piece of fresh fruit (sliced) and soy milk.

Soy yogurt with a piece of fresh fruit (sliced), pumpkin seeds, sunflower seeds and Golden Roasted Flaxseeds.

Rice cakes with almond butter and a mashed banana with a Revival Soy Shake.

Brown rice flakes soaked in soy milk with organic dried apricots (sliced), sunflower seeds, pumpkin seeds and Golden Roasted Flaxseeds.

Pancakes made with gluten-free flour and soy milk.

Fruit shake made with soy milk, berries, Golden Roasted Flaxseeds and ground almonds.

Lunch

A salad made from:
Jacket potato with a filling of your choice eg. salmon and chives, tuna and sweetcorn, baked beans, avocado or hummus.

Marinated tofu pieces.

Home-made soup, a wholesome snack or meal that is easy to make. Try incorporating soy milk.

Incorporate a combination of vegetables and beans and enhance with herbs and mild spices. Alternatively, you can buy very good organic ready-made soups from the supermarket, including gluten-free and dairy-free varieties.

Any form of protein, preferably oily fish, poultry or vegetarian alternatives like nuts, seeds, legumes, tofu and hummus.

Cheese, spinach and mushroom omelette made with soy milk.

Fruity, brown rice salad with dried apricots, sunflower and pumpkin seeds plus cheese or tuna.

Fresh fruit to follow.

Dinner

A good serving of protein – again, oily fish, poultry, game or vegetarian protein including tofu, plus three servings of vegetables, including one green variety like cabbage, spinach or broccoli.

Dessert

Fresh fruit salad with soy yogurt

Prune & tofu whip

Blackberry & rhubarb compote with Soy Dream or soy yogurt

Ginger fruit salad with soy yogurt

Raspberry & tofu brulée

Banana & rice pudding

Soy yogurt with chopped fruit and Roasted Flaxseeds

Beverages

Rooiboos (or Redbush) tea, a herbal tea with no caffeine and very little tannin.

Fruit herbal teas

Ground dandelion coffee or any caffeine-free alternatives

Fresh fruit juice

Carbonated water mixed with fruit juice

Organic fruit cordials

Nutritious Snacks

Natural soy yogurt with a handful of sunflower and pumpkin seeds

Revival Soy Shake, Crispy Bar or a soy smoothie

One or two slices of gluten-free bread or toast, or rice cakes with nut butter (almond, cashew and hazelnut are nutritious alternatives to peanut butter) or pure fruit spread

A slice of any wholesome gluten-free cake

Phyto Fix Bar

Dried fruit with sunflower and pumpkin seeds

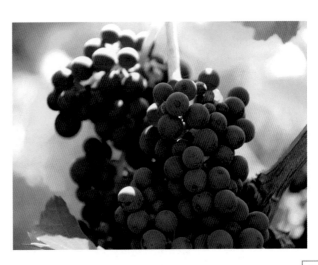

"After three months on the program, I have no pain or swollen joints in my hands or feet and I have no hot flashes during the day or night."

Jennifer Colby

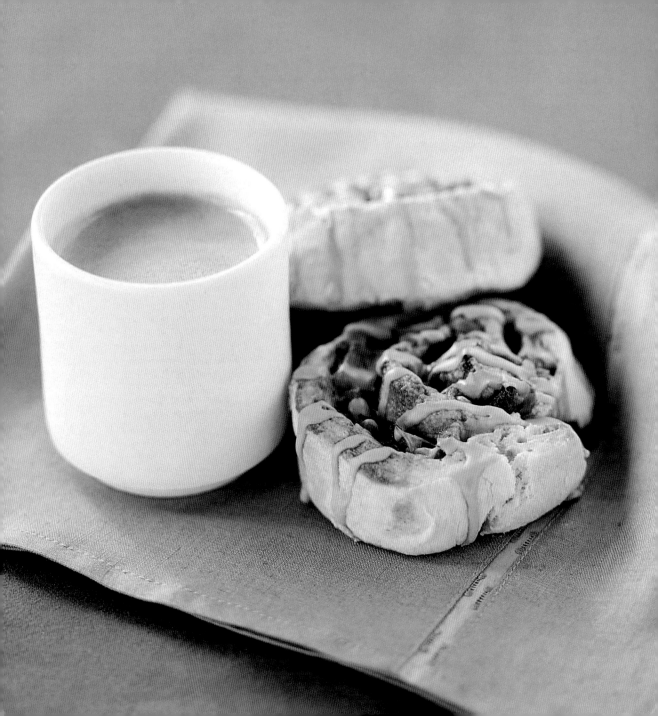

recipes

S oy-rich and phyto-rich food doesn't need to be bland or boring. Here is a selection of quick and easy recipes that are brimming with these essential nutrients and are guaranteed to tempt your taste buds. For a larger selection of delicious and nutritious recipes, visit our website at www.naturalmenopause.com.

Apple & Walnut Coffee Rolls
Makes 8

1¾oz butter
2 small Granny Smith apples, peeled, cored, diced
2¼oz (½ cup) walnuts, chopped
½ tsp ground cinnamon
3¼ oz (½ cup) brown sugar
12oz (2¼ cups) self-raising flour
1¹/₄ oz butter (extra), chopped
9floz (1 cup) soy milk

Icing
1 tsp instant coffee
1 tbsp hot water
3¼ oz (½ cup) icing sugar mixture

Preheat oven to 400°F (200°C). Line baking tray with baking paper. Heat butter in frying pan until foaming. Add apples and walnuts. Cook for 5 minutes or until apple softens. Add cinnamon and sugar, stirring over medium heat until sugar caramelises. Remove from heat and cool.

Place flour and extra butter in large mixing bowl and use your fingers to rub in butter until mixture resembles fine breadcrumbs. Make a well in the centre, add soy milk. Use a round-bladed knife in a cutting action to mix, forming a stiff dough. Use your hands to press dough into a ball. If dough is sticky, dust with a little flour. Place dough on a lightly floured surface and use your hands to press it into a 8inch x 12 inch (20cm x 30cm) rectangle. Spread apple mixture over dough, then quickly roll dough up to enclose filling. Place the roll seam-side down on a chopping board and cut into 8 equal pieces. Place cut-side up on prepared tray and bake for 20 minutes or until golden brown. Set aside to cool on a wire rack.

Icing
Combine coffee and water, then quickly stir through the icing sugar until the mixture is smooth. Drizzle over rolls with a teaspoon. Allow icing to set, then serve for a morning or afternoon treat.

281

Phyto Muesli
Makes 12 servings

1lb4oz (2½ cups) puffed rice
16oz (2 cups) cornflakes
4oz (½ cup) chopped almonds
4oz (½ cup) pumpkin seeds
4oz (½ cup) chopped pecans
4oz (½ cup) sesame seeds
4oz (½ cup) pine kernels
3oz (⅓ cup) organic flaxseeds
6oz (⅔ cup) organic raisins
4oz (½ cup) organic apricots, chopped

Mix all the ingredients together. Store in a sealed container. Serve with soy yogurt or soy milk and fresh fruit. Note: If you are constipated, sprinkle additional flaxseeds over your morning muesli.

Crunchy Almond Muesli
Serves 8

1lb (5 cups) rolled oats
4oz (½ cup) sunflower seeds
8oz (1½ cups) chopped almonds
¼ pint (⅝ cup) brown rice syrup
¼ pint (⅝ cup) soy oil
¼ pint (⅝ cup) unsweetened apple juice
8oz (1⅛ cups) raisins (preferably unsulphured)
4oz (½ cup) shredded coconut

Preheat oven to 300ºF (150ºC). Mix oats, seeds and almonds in a large bowl. Blend syrup, oil and juice in a jug and pour over mixture. Spread mixture onto baking tray and bake for 35 minutes until lightly browned, stirring every 5–10 minutes. Stir in raisins and coconut. Store in a sealed container. Serve with soy milk or yogurt.

Phyto Fruit Loaf
Makes 2 loaves

5oz (¾ cup) soy flour
4oz (½ cup) buckwheat flour
4oz (½ cup) flaxseeds (whole)
4oz (½ cup) ground almonds
2oz (¼ cup) sesame seeds
2oz (¼ cup) sunflower seeds
10oz (1⅓ cups) dried fruit
2 level tbsp unrefined superfine sugar
1 tsp nutmeg
1 tsp mixed spice
1 tbsp ground cinnamon
2 x 1in fresh ginger
2 tsp wheat-free baking powder
1½ pints (3 cups) soy milk

Mix all dry ingredients in a large bowl, then stir in the soy milk. Leave to stand for 1 hour. Spoon into 2 x 1lb prepared loaf tins. Bake at 350ºF (175ºC) for 60–90 minutes until firm on top. Transfer onto a wire rack and allow to cool. Serve warm or cold with butter, cheese, and fruit or nut spreads.

Phyto Sprinkle

4oz (½ cup) almonds
4oz (½ cup) sunflower seeds
4oz (½ cup) pumpkin seeds
4oz (½ cup) Golden Flaxseeds

Blend all ingredients to a coarse consistency. Store in a sealed container. This excellent source of phytoestrogens can easily be combined into your daily diet. Sprinkle over breakfast cereals, salads and desserts or use in bread and cake recipes.

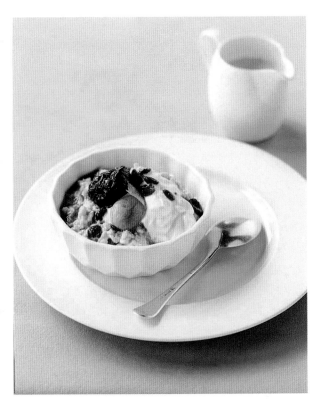

Winter Oatmeal with Spiced Dried Fruit Compote
Serves 4

9floz (1 cup) water
4oz (½ cup) superfine sugar
5½oz (1 cup) dried figs
4oz (½ cup) dried apricots
2oz (¼ cup) dried cranberries
2 cinnamon sticks
4 cloves
1 lemon
6½oz (2 cups) organic rolled oats
1¾ pints (4 cups) soy milk
Pinch of salt
4oz (½ cup) Greek yogurt

Bring water and sugar to a boil in a medium saucepan. Add dried fruit, cinnamon, cloves and 2 strips of lemon rind. Reduce heat and simmer for 10 minutes or until fruit is soft and plump. Juice the lemon and add to the pan. Set aside to cool slightly.

Place oats, soy milk and salt in a medium saucepan. Bring to a boil, then reduce heat to medium and cook for 10 minutes or until oatmeal thickens, stirring constantly. Serve with the fruit compote and yogurt.

Spanish Omelette
Serves 6

3 tbsp olive oil
3 small red potatoes (about 12oz), sliced
1 medium red bell pepper, cut into ¾in strips
1 red onion, halved, thinly sliced
2 bacon slices, rind trimmed, cut into strips
Salt & freshly ground black pepper
1 tbsp fresh oregano leaves
6 eggs
4floz (½ cup) soy milk
Salad of lettuce leaves, olives and shaved parmesan

Heat oil in a large, flameproof, non-stick frying pan over medium heat. Add potatoes and red bell pepper. Cover and cook for 10 minutes, stirring occasionally. Add onion and bacon. Cover and cook for a further 10 minutes, stirring occasionally. Season with salt and pepper. Add oregano.

Preheat grill on medium. Whisk together eggs and soy milk. Pour into pan. Cover and cook over medium heat for 5 minutes or until base is golden. Cook under preheated grill for a further 10 minutes or until top is golden. Slice and serve with salad.

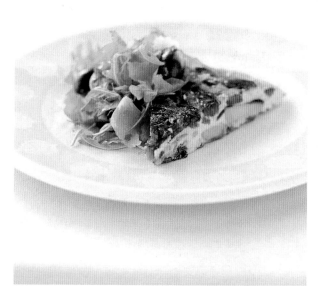

Chili & Corn Fritters with Scrambled Eggs
Serves 4

5½floz (1 cup) plain flour
1 tsp baking powder
Salt & freshly ground black pepper
2 corn cobs (or 1 cup corn niblets, drained, rinsed)
1 small red chili, finely chopped
2 eggs
4floz (½ cup) soy milk
2 tbsp vegetable oil
1¼oz (⅛ cup) baby spinach leaves
6 roma tomatoes, halved, grilled
6 slices prosciutto, grilled

Scrambled Eggs
4 eggs
2¼floz (¼ cup) soy milk
1¼oz butter

Fritters
Sift flour and baking powder into large bowl. Season with salt and pepper. Add corn, chili, eggs and soy milk. Mix to form a stiff batter. Heat oil in non-stick frying pan. Add 2 tablespoons of batter for each fritter. Cook for 2 minutes each side or until golden brown and cooked through. Drain on paper towel. Repeat until all batter is used.

Scrambled Eggs
Whisk eggs and soy milk. Season with salt and pepper. Heat butter in non-stick frying pan until foaming. Add egg mixture and cook over low heat, stirring occasionally, until just set. Serve eggs, spinach, tomato and prosciutto sandwiched between fritters.

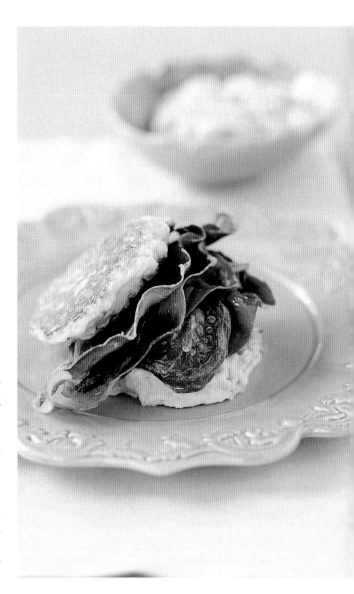

Banana Bread
Makes 1 loaf

2 ripe bananas, peeled
4floz (½ cup) vegetable oil
2 eggs, beaten
3¼oz (½ cup) brown sugar, lightly packed
4floz (½ cup) soy milk
8oz (1¼ cup) self-raising flour
3oz (½ cup) plain flour
1 tsp ground cinnamon
2¼oz (½ cup) roasted hazelnuts
4oz (½ cup) chopped dried banana
4¼oz (½ cup) fresh raspberries
Soy cream cheese and honey

Preheat oven to 350ºF (180°C). Lightly grease a 8½ in x 4¼in x 2½in (22cm x 11cm x 6cm) loaf pan. Mash bananas, then whisk together with oil, eggs, sugar and soy milk. Sift in flours and cinnamon. Gently fold through the wet ingredients with hazelnuts, dried banana and raspberries. Pour into prepared loaf pan and bake for 1 hour or until done. (Ready when a skewer inserted into centre comes out clean.) Slice and serve with cream cheese and honey.

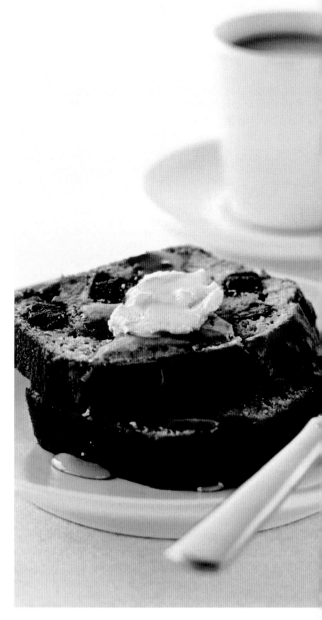

Apple Bread Rolls
Makes 12 rolls

4oz (½ cup) tofu
4oz (½ cup) grated apple
¼pint (¾ cup) soy milk
2 eggs
2oz (¼ cup) potato flour
2oz (¼ cup) corn meal
2oz (¼ cup) rice flour
2oz (¼ cup) soy flour
1 tsp baking soda
½ tsp cream of tartar
¼ tsp tartaric acid
1tbsp olive oil
2oz (¼ cup) soy margarine (for greasing tray)
1 tsp unrefined sugar

Preheat oven to 425ºF (220ºC). Beat tofu, apple, milk and eggs to a smooth puree. Mix dry ingredients with one tablespoon of olive oil, then fold into puree. (Do not over-mix or leave to stand, otherwise the dough will become heavy). Grease muffin tray with margarine and spoon in mixture. Bake for 12–15 minutes. Remove rolls from tray and cool. Serve hot with sweet or savoury dishes.

Note: As an alternative, try 4oz (½cup) of grated carrot in place of the tofu.

Soy and Rice Pancakes
Serves 4

2oz (¼ cup) soy flour
2oz (¼ cup) rice flour
1 small egg
½pint (1¼ cups) soy milk
Soy oil

Beat the flours, egg and milk into a thin batter. Wipe a little soy oil with greaseproof paper into a small, non-stick frying pan. Heat the oil until it starts to smoke. Pour about 2 tablespoons of batter into pan and swirl around to cover base. Cook for 60 seconds, then flip and briefly cook other side. Set aside. Repeat until you have used up all the batter. Makes 12 pancakes

Banana Oat Pancakes
Makes 12

2oz (¼ cup) oats
2oz (¼ cup) soy flour
1oz (⅛ cup) rice flour
1 tbsp baking powder
¼pint (¾ cups) unsweetened soy milk
2 bananas, thinly sliced

Combine dry ingredients in a bowl. Blend in milk to make a thin batter. Fold in banana. Pour some mixture into a lightly oiled, non-stick frying pan. Cook until bubbles appear on the surface, then flip and cook for about 1 minute. Serve warm with pure maple syrup, soy yogurt and fresh fruit.

Brown Rice and Watercress Salad
Serves 4

2oz (½ cup) brown rice, cooked
1 bunch watercress, washed and chopped
4oz (½ cup) sweetcorn, cooked and drained
1 green bell pepper, deseeded and chopped

Combine all ingredients. Season with black pepper.

Apple and Nut Salad
Serves 4

4 red apples, washed
Lemon juice
½ cucumber, thickly sliced and quartered
6 celery sticks, chopped
1 bunch of green onions, sliced
3oz (½ cup) natural peanuts

Core and roughly chop apples. Dip in lemon juice to slow discolouration. Combine all ingredients. Toss in the dressing of your choice.

Sweet Potato Salad
Serves 4

1lb (3 cups) sweet potato, steamed and cubed
1 tbsp soy oil
3 tbsp lemon juice
1-2 cloves garlic, crushed
1 tbsp parsley, chopped
1 tbsp basil, chopped
1 tbsp chives, chopped
1 tbsp spring onion, chopped

Combine all ingredients. Season with black pepper.

Nicoise Salad with Soy Milk Dressing
Serves 4

3 eggs
8 chat potatoes, halved
10½oz tuna steaks
Olive oil spray
7oz (¾ cup) baby beans
7oz (¾ cup) grape tomatoes, halved
4oz (½ cup) small black olives
1 baby cos lettuce, leaves separated

Dressing
5½oz (¾ cup) silken tofu
3½floz (½ cup) soy milk
1 clove garlic, chopped
1 tsp Dijon mustard
2 tbsp lime juice

Place eggs in small saucepan and cover with cold water. Bring to a boil, then reduce heat to low and simmer for 5 minutes. Refresh in cold water, then peel and set aside.

Cook potatoes in boiling salted water for 10 minutes or until just cooked. Lightly spray tuna with olive oil, then chargrill for 2–3 minutes each side or until just cooked. Flake into pieces using 2 forks. Blanch beans in boiling salted water for 1 minute, then refresh in cold water. Toss eggs, potatoes, tuna, beans, tomatoes, olives and lettuce together in a large bowl.

Dressing
Combine all ingredients in a blender until smooth. Season with salt and freshly ground black pepper. Drizzle over salad.

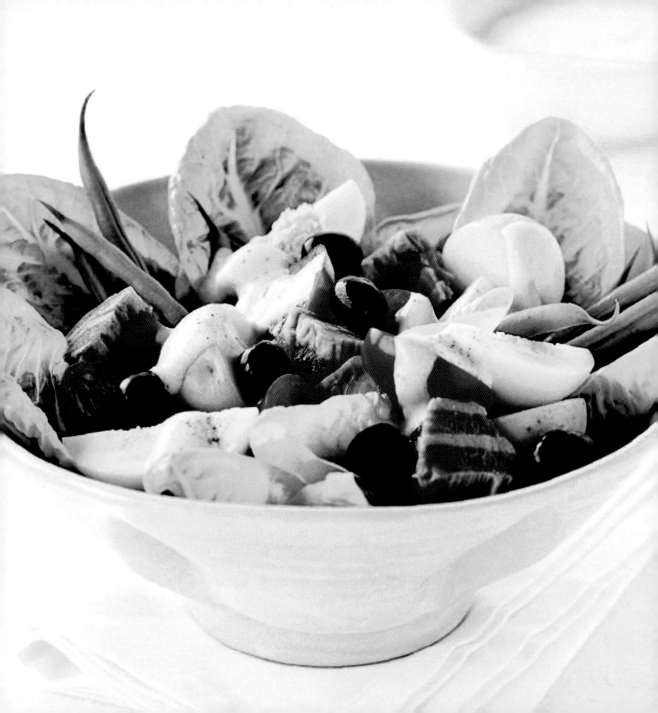

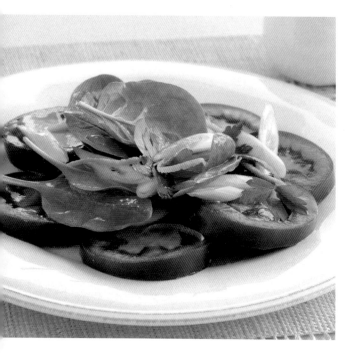

Apple, Celery and Beetroot Salad
Serves 4

1 large beetroot, cooked and cubed
1 apple, sliced, skin left on
1 tbsp French dressing
1 stick celery, diced
1 tbsp chopped walnuts
Combine all ingredients.

Watercress Soup
Serves 4

2oz (¼ cup) soy margarine
1 medium onion, finely chopped
8oz potatoes, peeled and diced
1 pint (2¼ cups) vegetable stock
pinch of nutmeg
4 bunches of watercress, washed and trimmed
black pepper to taste

Melt the margarine in a frying pan, add the onion and fry gently for about 5 minutes or until onion is transparent. Add the potato, vegetable stock and nutmeg and simmer for 15 minutes. Add the watercress and simmer for a further 10 minutes. Purée the soup in a blender or food processor, then push through a sieve. Add black pepper to taste and serve .

Orange and Avocado Salad
Serves 2

2 tomatoes
2 oranges
1 green onion, finely chopped
2 tbsp lemon juice
2 tbsp orange juice
2 tsp flaxseed oil
¼ tsp chopped fresh ginger
lettuce leaves

Slice tomatoes. Mix with orange pieces and onion. Mix juices, oil and ginger, then pour over salad. Serve on lettuce leaves or on its own.

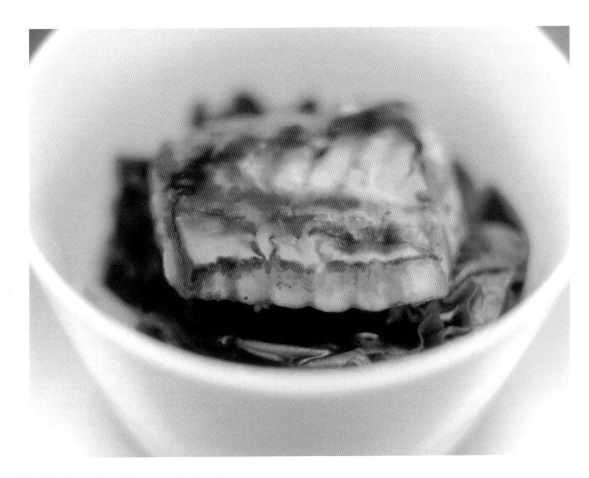

Fish with Sweet Soy Sauce on Spinach
Serves 2

2 x 6½oz fish fillets
1 tsp sesame oil
2 tbsp sweet soy sauce
9floz (1 cup) chicken stock
4 bunches spinach leaves
2 cloves garlic, chopped
1 red chili, chopped
1 tbsp wheat-free tamari

Sear each side of the fish in a hot pan with sesame oil for 2–3 minutes until just done, adding a little stock if necessary. Add soy sauce and ½ cup stock. Heat through until fish has been glazed by the sauce. Meanwhile, stir-fry the spinach with the garlic, chili, tamari and remaining stock until spinach wilts, then place in bowls and top with the fish.

Corn Chowder with Garlic Shrimps
Serves 2

1¼oz butter
1 small onion, finely diced
3 garlic cloves, finely chopped
1 medium potato, peeled, diced
2 corn cobs (or 1 cup corn niblets, drained, rinsed)
1 celery stick, diced
1¼pint (3 cups) soy milk
1 vegetable bullion cube, crumbled
Freshly ground black pepper
1 tbsp olive oil
9oz (1 cup) peeled green shrimps
½ cup fresh flat-leaf parsley leaves

Heat butter in large saucepan until foaming. Add onion and one-third of garlic. Cook over medium heat for 2 minutes. Add potato. Cook for 2 minutes. Add corn, celery and soy milk. Bring to a boil, then reduce heat and simmer for 10 minutes or until vegetables are just tender. Add stock and pepper.

Heat oil in a frying pan. Add remaining garlic and shrimps. Cook over medium-high heat for 2 minutes or until shrimps are just cooked. Remove from heat and stir through parsley. Spoon chowder into bowls and serve topped with shrimps.

Chicken Noodle Soup
Serves 4

3½pints (8 cups) chicken stock
2 cloves garlic, chopped
1 tbsp ginger, grated
2 sticks lemongrass, finely chopped
2 chicken breasts, skinless
9oz (1cup) shiitaki mushrooms
1 head broccoli, cut into flowerets
9oz (1cup) packet dried soba noodles

Combine stock, garlic, ginger and lemongrass in a large saucepan and bring to a boil. Add chicken and gently simmer for 8–10 minutes until cooked through. Add mushrooms and broccoli and simmer for a further 3–5 minutes. Meanwhile, cook noodles in plenty of boiling water until al dente, then drain and divide into serving bowls. Remove chicken from soup and slice, then return it to soup and stir through. Ladle soup over noodles and serve.

Note: As an alternative, substitute soba noodles with rice noodles, which are wheat-free and gluten-free.

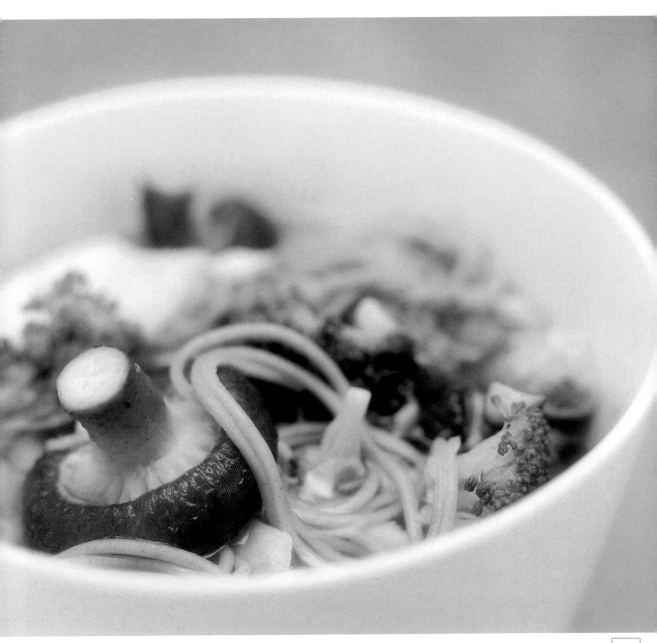

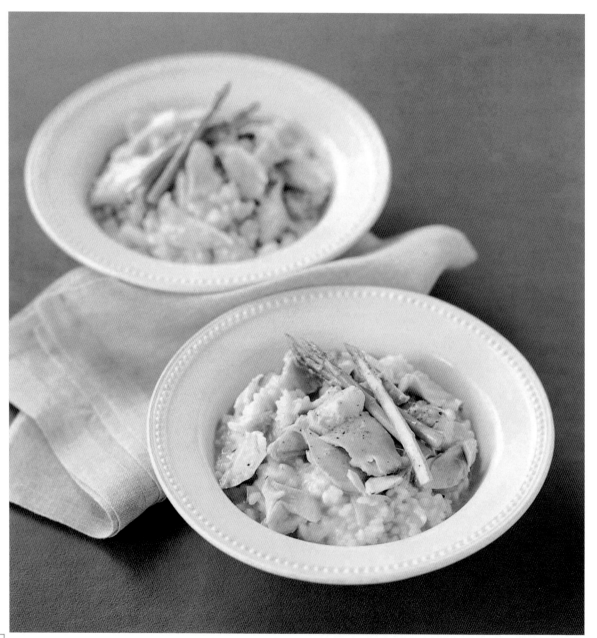

Preserved Lemon Risotto
with Flaked Salmon & Asparagus
Serves 6

1¼pints (3 cups) soy milk
18floz (2 cups) chicken stock
1¼oz butter
1 tbsp olive oil
1 small red onion, thinly sliced
2 garlic cloves, finely chopped
½ preserved lemon, chopped
11½oz (1½ cups) arborio rice
Salt & freshly ground black pepper
10½oz marinated artichoke hearts, sliced
14oz salmon fillet
Olive oil, for rubbing
1 bunch asparagus, trimmed

Place soy milk and stock in a saucepan and bring just to a boil. Reduce heat to a simmer. Heat butter and oil in a saucepan over medium heat. Fry onion and garlic until soft, stirring often. Add lemon and rice. Stir over medium heat for 1–2 minutes until the rice grains are slightly glassy.

Slowly add soy milk and stock to rice, stirring constantly until liquid is completely absorbed. Continue to add liquid, a ladle at a time, stirring constantly until absorbed. Continue stirring until rice is just cooked. (This process should take about 20 minutes.) Season with salt and pepper. Stir through artichokes. Set aside while you cook salmon.

Season the salmon with salt and pepper, then rub with olive oil. Cook salmon over medium heat for 2–3 minutes per side until just cooked. Transfer to a plate and use two forks to gently flake into pieces. Blanch asparagus in boiling water, then drain and refresh under cold running water. Serve risotto topped with salmon and asparagus.

Green Chicken Curry
Serves 6

1 tbsp vegetable oil
1lb2oz chicken tenderloins, cut into strips
2-3 tbsp Thai green curry paste
¼pint can coconut cream
9floz (1 cup) soy milk
1 tbsp fish sauce
8oz can sliced bamboo shoots, rinsed
4½oz (¾cup) baby corn
4oz (½cup) snow peas, trimmed
4oz (½ cup) fresh Thai basil leaves
Steamed jasmine rice

Heat the oil, add chicken and curry paste. Cook over medium heat, stirring constantly for 5 minutes or until seared all over. Add coconut cream, soy milk and fish sauce. Bring to a boil, stirring occasionally. Add bamboo shoots and corn. Cook until corn is just tender. Remove from heat and stir in snow peas and basil. Serve with rice.

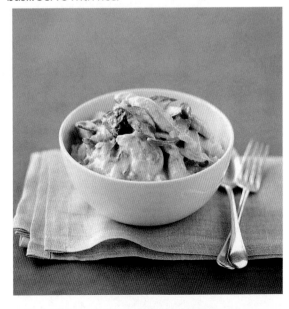

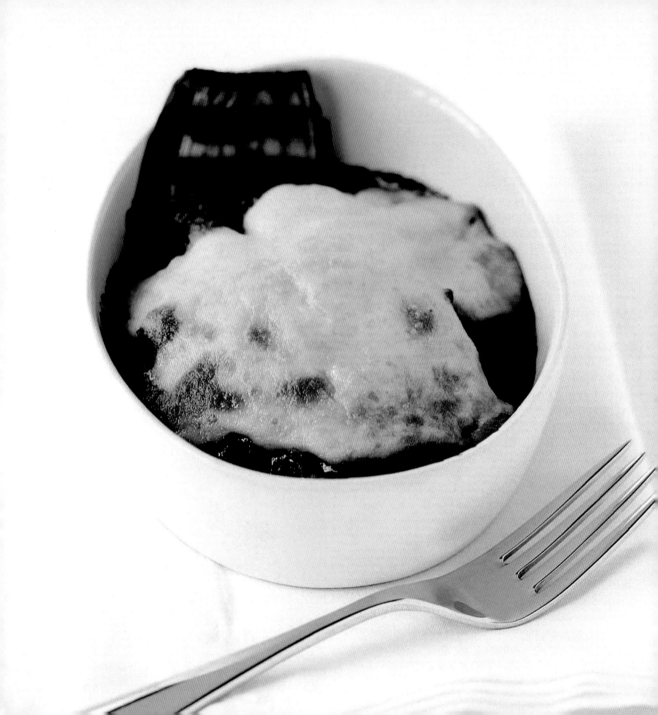

Individual Moussaka
Serves 6

1 aubergine, trimmed and sliced lengthways
into 6 thin slices
Olive oil spray

Meat Sauce
1 tbsp olive oil
1 onion, diced
2 cloves garlic, chopped
1lb2oz ground beef
1 tbsp chopped fresh oregano
½ tsp ground cinnamon
13floz (1½ cups) tomato purée
4floz (½ cup) red wine
1 tsp white sugar

White Sauce
2¼oz butter
2 tbsp plain flour
13floz (1½ cups) soy milk
1 egg, beaten

Preheat oven to 350°F (180°C). Lightly spray aubergine slices with oil and chargrill for 1 minute each side or until soft and charred. Set aside.

Meat Sauce
Heat oil in frying pan over medium heat. Sauté onion and garlic for 3 minutes or until soft. Add beef. Toss until beef browns. Stir in oregano, cinnamon, tomato and wine. Reduce heat to low and simmer for 20 minutes or until sauce is thick. Season with salt and pepper, and the sugar.

White Sauce
Meanwhile, melt butter in small saucepan over medium heat. Add flour and stir for 1–2 minutes using a wooden spoon. Gradually add soy milk while stirring until sauce comes to a boil. Remove pan from heat and season, then whisk in the egg.

To assemble moussaka, lay a slice of aubergine in 6 separate 9floz (1 cup) baking dishes. Divide meat sauce between 6 dishes and top with white sauce. Bake for 15 minutes or until golden brown. Serve warm with a salad.

Hummus
Serves 4

8oz (1 cup) chick peas
5½oz (½ cup) sesame seeds
2 tbsp tahini
2 tbsp soy oil
5 cloves garlic
3 lemons

Soak chick peas overnight in water. Drain and wash. Place in a pot of water and bring to a boil, then simmer gently for 2 hours until tender. Drain again. Blend seeds, tahini, oil, garlic and half the lemon juice to a smooth puree. Gradually add chick peas and remaining lemon juice, blending until smooth. If desired, add a pinch of paprika for a touch of spiciness. Serve with rice cakes.

Cauliflower Soup
Serves 4

2oz (¼cup) soy margarine
4oz (½cup) soy flour
9floz (1cup) soy milk
1½pint (3¾cups) vegetable stock
1 large cauliflower, broken into florets
1 tsp dried chervil

Melt margarine in large saucepan. Add flour and cook for 1 minute, stirring constantly. Remove from heat and gradually stir in milk and stock until smooth. Add cauliflower and chervil. Season with black pepper. Simmer gently for 15 minutes until cauliflower is just soft. Blend to a smooth puree. Serve piping hot with crusty bread.

Salmon Steaks with Ginger
Serves 2

2 salmon steaks
2 tbsp lemon juice
1in cube of ginger, peeled and finely chopped

Preheat oven to 350°F (180°C). Place each salmon steak on a piece of foil. Add half the lemon juice and ginger to each steak. Season with black pepper. Wrap steaks individually in foil and bake for 20 minutes. Serve with vegetables or salad.

Tofu, Bean and Herb Stir-fry
Serves 4

2 tbsp soy oil
10oz (12 ¼ cups) tofu, drained, dried, cubed
2 garlic cloves, crushed
12oz (1½ cups) green beans
3 tbsp chopped fresh herbs (thyme, parsley, chives, chervil)
4 green onions, thinly sliced
2 tbsp tamari sauce

Heat 1 tbsp of soy oil in a frying pan or wok. Add tofu and garlic and stir fry for 2 minutes. Lift tofu out with a slotted spoon and drain. Heat remaining oil, then add beans and stir fry gently for 4–5 minutes. Add remaining ingredients and stir fry a further minute. Return tofu to pan and heat for 1 minute. Serve immediately with rice or noodles.

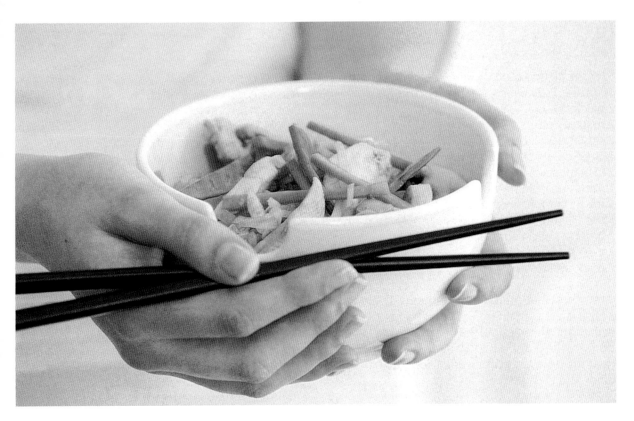

Noodles in Spicy Sesame Sauce
Serves 4

1lb (2¼ cups) rice noodles
¼pint (⅝ cup) sesame oil
3 cloves garlic, finely chopped
2 tbsp fresh ginger, finely grated
5 spring onions, finely chopped
1 tsp chili powder
¼pint (⅝ cup) tahini
2 tbsp tamari sauce
3 tbsp rice vinegar
1 tbsp tomato puree
¼pint (⅝ cup) cold water
1 large tomato, finely chopped

Bring a large pot of salted water to a boil. Drop in noodles and cook for about 15 minutes. Heat oil in a saucepan and sauté garlic and ginger for 3 minutes, stirring constantly. Add onions and stir a further 3 minutes. Season with black pepper. Add chili powder and stir for 1 minute. Mix the remaining ingredients (except chopped tomato) together and add to saucepan. Stir well and simmer. Place noodles on a serving dish and spoon sauce over top. Garnish with chopped tomato.

Jacket Potatoes With Spicy Soya Beans
Serves 6

6 large baking potatoes, scrubbed and scored
16oz dried soy beans, washed and drained
3 bay leaves
2 tbsp soy oil
2 cloves garlic, chopped
1 large onion, chopped
2 inch piece of cinnamon
10oz (1¼ cups) tomato purée
5floz (⅔ cup) molasses
5 floz (⅔ cup) prepared mustard
2 pints (4 cups) vegetable stock
2 tbsp cider vinegar
1 tbsp tamari sauce

Wash the beans and soak overnight. Drain, rinse well and drain again before cooking for 2–3 hours with the bay leaves until the beans are soft. Remove from the heat and drain away the cooking water. Heat the oil in a saucepan and sauté the garlic and onion until tender.

Add the cinnamon and stir for 1 minute. Add the tomato purée, molasses, mustard and stock, stir well and bring to the boil. Add the beans, bring to the boil again then cover the pan, reduce the heat to low and simmer gently for 1 hour. Stir once during this time, adding more stock if necessary.

At the end of the cooking time, stir in the vinegar and soy sauce. Remove the pot from the heat and serve immediately. The beans should be thick and the sauce richly flavoured. Spoon over potatoes and serve.

Potatoes
Preheat the oven to 400ºF (200ºC). Bake the potatoes for about 45 minutes, or until tender.

Rosemary Arancini
Makes 12

18floz (2 cups) soy milk
18floz (2 cups) chicken stock
1¼oz (¼ cup) butter
1 onion, finely diced
1 clove garlic, crushed
8oz (1 cup) arborio rice
2¼oz (¼ cup) mozzarella, cut into cubes
Oil, for deep-frying
2 eggs, beaten
8oz (1 cup) dry breadcrumbs
12 small sprigs fresh rosemary

Pour soy milk and stock into medium-sized saucepan and bring to a boil. Remove from heat and set aside to cool.

Heat butter in large saucepan. Sauté onion and garlic over medium heat for 2–3 minutes or until soft. Add rice and stir for 1 minute or until rice is clear. Gradually ladle soy milk and stock into rice mixture, stirring with wooden spoon. Continue adding liquid, one ladle at a time, each time waiting for liquid to be absorbed before adding more. (This process should take about 20 minutes). Set risotto aside to cool.

Divide risotto into 12 equal portions and roll into balls using your palms. Gently press your thumb into each ball and place in a cube of mozzarella, then pinch risotto to enclose cheese and roll again. Place balls on a tray, cover and refrigerate until required.

Heat oil in small frying pan until hot. (Oil is ready when a small cube of bread turns golden in 1–2 minutes). Dip balls, one at a time, first into beaten egg, then into breadcrumbs. Spear each ball with a sprig of rosemary and deep-fry, two at a time, until golden brown. Use a slotted spoon to transfer cooked balls onto paper towel. Serve warm.

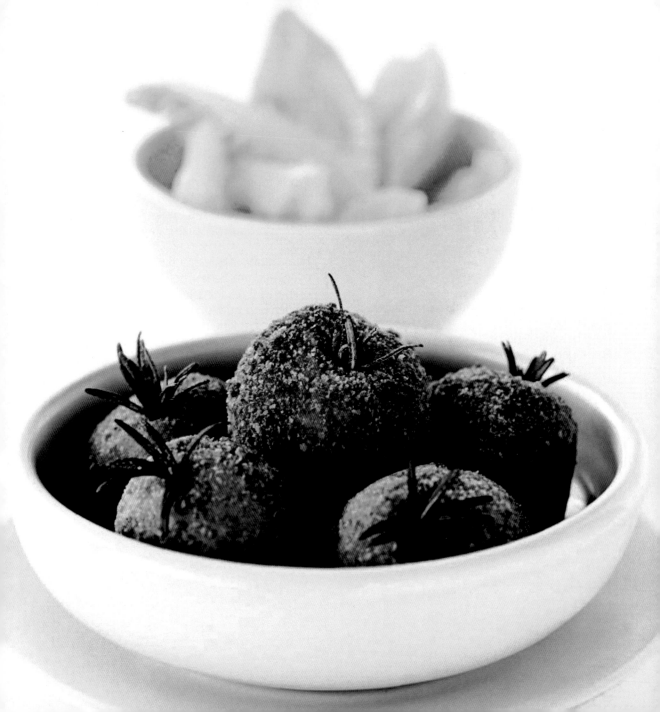

Strawberry Soufflé Pancakes
Serves 4

9floz (1 cup) soy milk
2 eggs, separated
3 tsp grated lemon rind
5½oz (1 cup) self-raising flour
1 tsp vanilla essence
1 tbsp superfine sugar
Pinch of salt
¾oz butter
1lb (2½cups) strawberries, hulled and halved
3 tbsp honey
1 tbsp balsamic vinegar
Icing sugar

Whisk together soy milk, egg yolks, lemon rind, flour, superfine sugar, vanilla and salt. In a dry bowl, whisk egg whites until stiff peaks form. Gently fold egg whites through pancake batter.

Heat butter, a little at a time, in non-stick frying pan over medium heat. Cook large spoonfuls of batter, one at a time, for a few minutes each side or until golden and puffed. Transfer pancakes to a plate and continue cooking remaining batter. Toss strawberries with honey and vinegar. Serve with warm pancakes. Dust with a little icing sugar.

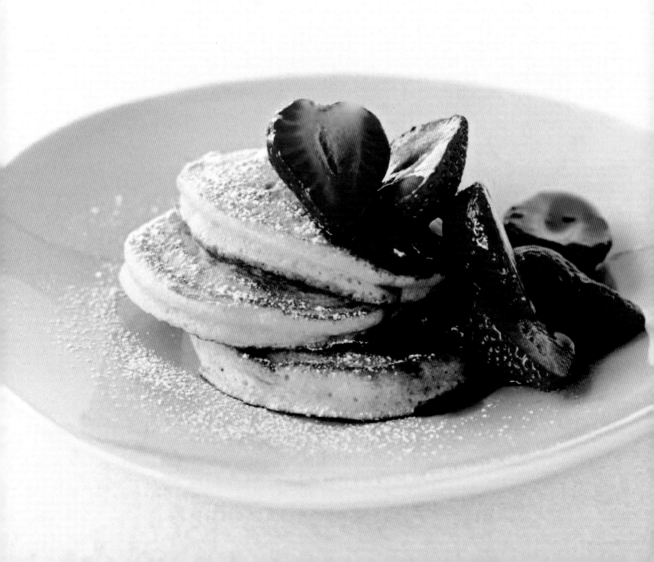

Prune and Tofu Dessert
Serves 4

4oz (½ cup) prunes (preferably unsulphured)
8oz (1 cup) tofu
2 tbsp natural maple syrup or honey

Soak prunes overnight. Drain, place in a saucepan and cover with water. Simmer for 10–15 minutes until really tender. Drain again (reserving the liquid). Blend prunes well with tofu and syrup. Add just enough cooking liquor to make a thick, soft puree. Pour into sundae glasses and chill until ready to serve.

Banana and Rice Pudding
Serves 4

1lb (2 cups) mashed banana
7oz (1cup) uncooked brown rice
1¼pint (3cups) soy milk
1 tsp pure vanilla essence
rind of 1 lemon
1 tsp nutmeg

Preheat oven to 350°F (180ºC). Place all ingredients (except nutmeg) in a casserole dish and stir well. Sprinkle nutmeg over top. (Use a tea strainer to sprinkle evenly). Bake for 1½–2 hours. Serve on its own or with stewed fruit. .

Banana Shake
Serves 4

4 very ripe bananas
1¾pints (4cups) soy milk, chilled
2oz (¼cup) ground almonds
¼ tsp ground nutmeg

Blend all ingredients well. Serve chilled.

Rhubarb and Blueberry Smoothie
Serves 4

1lb (2 cups) rhubarb, washed and trimmed
1lb (2 cups) blueberries, washed
1¾pint (4 cups) soy milk, chilled
20 ice cubes, crushed
¼ tsp vanilla essence

Blend all ingredients well. Serve chilled with extra ice if desired.

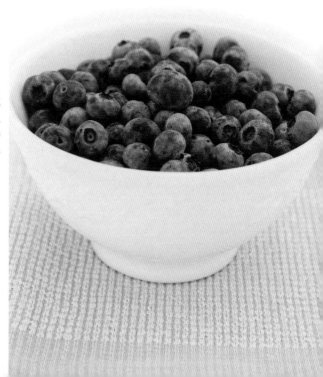

Raspberry and Tofu Brulée
Serves 4

7oz (1cup) raspberries
9oz (1¼cup)) silken tofu
2 tbsp honey
3 tbsp soft brown sugar

Blend raspberries, tofu and honey until smooth. Pour into 4 ramekins. Sprinkle sugar on top and grill until sugar forms a hard, golden layer.

Chewy Fruit Bars
Makes 12–16 bars

4oz (½cups) dried apricots, unsulphured, diced
1 tsp grated orange rind
3½floz (½cup) orange juice
2oz (¼cup) almonds, chopped
2oz (¼cup) shredded coconut
2oz (¼cup) puffed rice
4oz (½cup) ground almonds
2oz (¼cup) dried fruit (raisins, apple, peach), chopped
extra shredded coconut

Simmer apricots and rind in orange juice for 5 minutes until soft. Toast almonds in oven or under grill. Toast coconut the same way, making sure it doesn't burn. Blend apricot mixture, coconut, puffed rice and ground almonds. (This mixture is quite sticky, so stop the blender and scrape it from the sides once or twice). Pour mixture into a bowl and add toasted almonds and dried fruit. Mix by hand into a large ball. Line a baking tray with foil and sprinkle with extra coconut. Flatten out the mixture and sprinkle with more coconut. Cut into bars and allow to dry (preferably overnight) before storing in a sealed container. Use within 1 week.

Phyto Fix Bars
Makes 8 bars

2oz (¼cup) sesame seeds
4oz (½cup) Golden Flaxseeds
2oz (¼cup) sunflower seeds
2oz (¼cup) pumpkin seeds
4oz (½cup) vine fruits (sultanas, raisins, currants)
2oz (¼cup) dried apricots, chopped
3oz (¾cup) soy protein isolate
4oz (½cup) puffed rice
2 tsp mixed spice
2 tsp ginger powder (optional)
4oz (½cup) date syrup
2oz (¼cup) ginger or rice syrup
¼pint (⅝cup) soy milk

Preheat oven to 350°F (180°C). Mix dry ingredients in a bowl. Add syrup and milk and mix thoroughly. Grease a Swiss roll baking tin. Pour in mixture and smooth the surface. Bake for 20 minutes. Allow to cool, then cut into bars.

"If you do a moderate amount of exercise -
20 minutes every day - it actually lowers your rate of hot flashes...
and improves your bones."

Dr Sally Hope

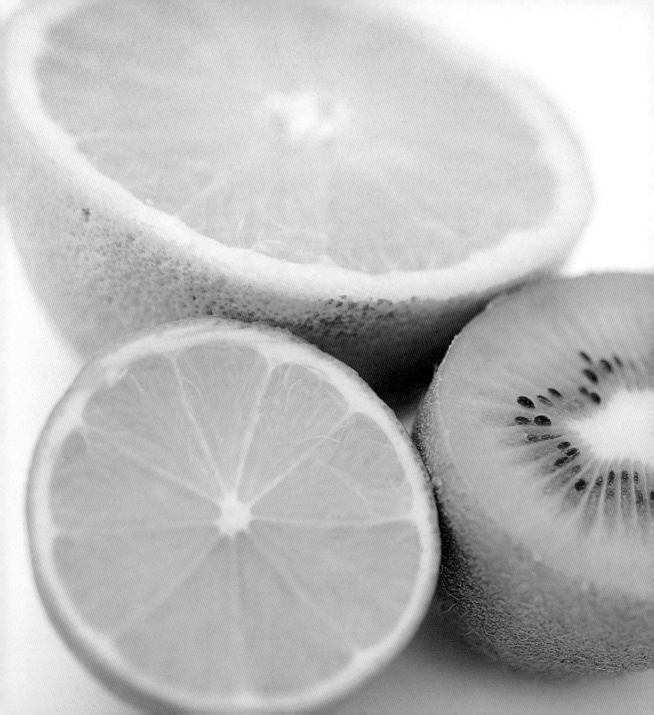

nutrient content of food

Unless otherwise stated, foods listed are raw.

Vitamin A – Retinol
Micrograms per 100g (3.5oz)

Non-fat milk	1
2% reduced fat milk	21
Grilled herring	49
Full cream milk	52
Oatmeal made with milk	56
Cheddar cheese	325
Margarine	800
Butter	815
Lamb's liver	15,000

Vitamin B1 – Thiamin
Milligrams per 100 g (3.5oz)

Peaches	0.02
Cottage cheese	0.02
Cox's apple	0.03
Full cream milk	0.04
Non-fat milk	0.04
2% reduced fat milk	0.04
Cheddar cheese	0.04
Bananas	0.04
White grapes	0.04
French beans	0.04
Low-fat yogurt	0.05
Cantaloupe melon	0.05
Tomato	0.06
Green bell peppers, raw	0.07
Boiled egg	0.08
Roast chicken	0.08

Grilled cod	0.08
Haddock, steamed	0.08
Roast turkey	0.09
Mackerel, cooked	0.09
Savoy cabbage, boiled	0.10
Oranges	0.10
Brussels sprouts	0.10
Potatoes, new, boiled	0.11
Soy beans, boiled	0.12
Red bell peppers, raw	0.12
Lentils, boiled	0.14
Steamed salmon	0.20
Corn	0.20
White spaghetti, boiled	0.21
Almonds	0.24
White self-raising flour	0.30
Plaice, steamed	0.30
Bacon, cooked	0.35
Walnuts	0.40
Wholemeal flour	0.47
Lamb's kidney	0.49
Brazil nuts	1.00
Corn flakes	1.00
Rice Krispies	1.00
Wheatgerm	2.01

Vitamin B2 – Riboflavin
Milligrams per 100 g (3.5oz)

Cabbage, boiled	0.01
Potatoes, boiled	0.01
Brown rice, boiled	0.02
Pear	0.03
Cooked w/meal spaghetti	0.03

White self-raising flour	0.03
Orange	0.04
Spinach, cooked	0.05
Baked beans	0.06
Banana	0.06
White bread	0.06
Green bell peppers, raw	0.08
Lentils, boiled	0.08
Hovis	0.09
Soy beans, boiled	0.09
Wholemeal bread	0.09
Wholemeal flour	0.09
Peanuts	0.10
Baked salmon	0.11
Red bell peppers, raw	0.15
Full cream milk	0.17
Avocado	0.18
Grilled herring	0.18
2% reduced fat milk	0.18
Roast chicken	0.19
Roast turkey	0.21
Cottage cheese	0.26
Soy flour	0.31
Boiled shrimps	0.34
Boiled egg	0.35
Topside of beef, cooked	0.35
Leg of lamb, cooked	0.38
Cheddar cheese	0.40
Muesli	0.70
Almonds	0.75
Corn flakes	1.50
Rice Krispies	1.50

Vitamin B3 – Niacin
Milligrams per 100g (3.5oz)

Boiled egg	0.07
Cheddar cheese	0.07
Full cream milk	0.08
Non-fat milk	0.09
2% reduced fat milk	0.09
Cottage cheese	0.13
Cox's apple	0.20
Cabbage, boiled	0.30
Orange	0.40
Baked beans	0.50
Potatoes, boiled	0.50
Soy beans, boiled	0.50
Lentils, boiled	0.60
Banana	0.70
Tomato	1.00
Avocado	1.10
Green bell peppers, raw	1.10
Brown rice	1.30
Cooked w/meal spaghetti	1.30
White self-raising flour	1.50
Grilled cod	1.70
White bread	1.70
Soy flour	2.00
Red bell peppers, raw	2.20
Almonds	3.10
Grilled herring	4.00
Wholemeal bread	4.10
Hovis	4.20
Wholemeal flour	5.70
Muesli	6.50
Topside of beef, cooked	6.50
Leg of lamb, cooked	6.60
Baked salmon	7.00
Roast chicken	8.20
Roast turkey	8.50
Boiled shrimps	9.50
Peanuts	13.80
Rice Krispies	16.00
Corn flakes	16.00

Vitamin B6 – Pyridoxine
Milligrams per 100g (3.5oz)

Carrots	0.05
Full cream milk	0.06
Non-fat milk	0.06
2% reduced fat milk	0.06
Satsuma	0.07
White bread	0.07
White rice	0.07
Cabbage, boiled	0.08
Cottage cheese	0.08
Cox's apple	0.08
Wholemeal pasta	0.08
Frozen peas	0.09
Spinach, boiled	0.09
Cheddar cheese	0.10
Orange	0.10
Broccoli	0.11
Hovis	0.11
Baked beans	0.12
Boiled egg	0.12
Red kidney beans, cooked	0.12
Wholemeal bread	0.12
Tomatoes	0.14
Almonds	0.15
Cauliflower	0.15
Brussels sprouts	0.19
Sweet corn, boiled	0.21
Leg of lamb, cooked	0.22
Grapefruit juice	0.23
Roast chicken	0.26
Lentils, boiled	0.28
Banana	0.29
Brazil nuts	0.31
Potatoes, boiled	0.32
Roast turkey	0.33
Grilled herring	0.33
Topside of beef, cooked	0.33
Avocado	0.36
Grilled cod	0.38
Baked salmon	0.57
Soy flour	0.57
Hazelnuts	0.59
Peanuts	0.59
Walnuts	0.67
Muesli	1.60
Corn flakes	1.80
Rice Krispies	1.80
Special K	2.20

Vitamin B12 – Cyanocobalamine
Micrograms per 100g (3.5oz)

Tempeh	0.10
Miso	0.20
Quorn	0.30
Full cream milk	0.40
Non-fat milk	0.40
2% reduced fat milk	0.40
Cottage cheese	0.70
Choux buns	1.00
Eggs, boiled	1.00
Eggs, poached	1.00
Halibut, steamed	1.00
Lobster, boiled	1.00
Sponge cake	1.00
Turkey, white meat	1.00
Waffles	1.00
Cheddar cheese	1.20
Eggs, scrambled	1.20
Squid	1.30
Eggs, fried	1.60
Shrimps, boiled	1.80
Parmesan cheese	1.90
Beef, lean	2.00
Cod, baked	2.00

Corn flakes	2.00	
Pork, cooked	2.00	
Raw beef, ground	2.00	
Rice Krispies	2.00	
Steak, lean, grilled	2.00	
Edam cheese	2.10	
Eggs, whole, battery	2.40	
Milk, powdered, full cream	2.40	
Milk, powdered, non-fat	2.60	
Eggs, whole, free-range	2.70	
Kambu seaweed	2.80	
Squid, frozen	2.90	
Taramasalata	2.90	
Duck, cooked	3.00	
Turkey, dark meat	3.00	
Grapenuts	5.00	
Tuna in oil	5.00	
Herring, cooked	6.00	
Herring roe, fried	6.00	
Steamed salmon	6.00	
Mackerel, fried	10.0	
Rabbit, stewed	10.0	
Cod's roe, fried	11.0	
Oysters, raw	15.0	
Nori seaweed	27.5	
Sardines in oil	28.0	
Lamb's kidney, fried	79.0	

Folate/Folic Acid
Micrograms per 100g (3.5oz)

Cox's apple	4.0
Leg of lamb, cooked	4.0
Full cream milk	6.0
Non-fat milk	6.0
2% reduced fat milk	6.0
Oatmeal with 2% reduced fat milk	7.0
Turnip, baked	8.0
Sweet potato, boiled	8.0
Cucumber	9.0

Grilled herring	10.0
Roast chicken	10.0
Avocado	11.0
Grilled cod	12.0
Banana	14.0
Roast turkey	15.0
Carrots	17.0
Sweet potato	17.0
Tomatoes	17.0
Topside of beef, cooked	17.0
Swede, boiled	18.0
Strawberries	20.0
Brazil nuts	21.0
Red bell peppers, raw	21.0
Green bell peppers, raw	23.0
Rye bread	24.0
Dates, fresh	25.0
New potatoes, boiled	25.0
Grapefruit	26.0
Oatcakes	26.0
Cottage cheese	27.0
Baked salmon	29.0
Cabbage, boiled	29.0
Onions, boiled	29.0
White bread	29.0
Orange	31.0
Baked beans	33.0
Cheddar cheese	33.0
Clementines	33.0
Raspberries	33.0
Satsuma	33.0
Blackberries	34.0
Rye crispbread	35.0
Potato, baked in skin	36.0
Radish	38.0
Boiled egg	39.0
Hovis	39.0
Wholemeal bread	39.0
Red kidney beans, boiled	42.0

Potato, baked	44.0
Frozen peas	47.0
Almonds	48.0
Parsnips, boiled	48.0
Cauliflower	51.0
Green beans, boiled	57.0
Broccoli	64.0
Walnuts	66.0
Artichoke	68.0
Hazelnuts	72.0
Spinach, boiled	90.0
Brussels sprouts	110.0
Peanuts	110.0
Muesli	140.0
Sweet corn, boiled	150.0
Asparagus	155.0
Chickpeas	180.0
Lamb's liver, fried	240.0
Corn flakes	250.0
Rice Krispies	250.0
Calf's liver, fried	320.0

Vitamin C
Milligrams per 100g (3.5oz)

Full cream milk	1.00
Non-fat milk	1.00
Red kidney beans	1.00
Carrots	2.00
Cucumber	2.00
Muesli with dried fruit	2.00
Apricots, raw	6.00
Avocado	6.00
Pear	6.00
Potato, boiled	6.00
Spinach, boiled	8.00
Cox's apple	9.00
Turnip	10.00
Banana	11.0
Frozen peas	12.0

Lamb's liver, fried	12.0
Pineapple	12.0
Powdered milk, non-fat	13.0
Gooseberries	14.0
Raw dates	14.0
Melon	17.0
Tomatoes	17.0
Cabbage, boiled	20.0
Canteloupe melon	26.0
Cauliflower	27.0
Satsuma	27.0
Peach	31.0
Raspberries	32.0
Bran flakes	35.0
Grapefruit	36.0
Mangoes	37.0
Nectarine	37.0
Cumquats	39.0
Broccoli	44.0
Lychees	45.0
Unsweetened apple juice	49.0
Orange	54.0
Kiwi fruit	59.0
Brussels sprouts	60.0
Strawberries	77.0
Blackcurrants	115.0

Vitamin D

Micrograms per 100g (3.5oz)

Non-fat milk	0.01
Full cream milk	0.03
Fromage frais	0.05
Cheddar cheese	0.26
Corn flakes	2.80
Rice Krispies	2.80
Kellogg's Start	4.20
Margarine	8.00

Vitamin E

Milligrams per 100g (3.5oz)

2% reduced fat milk	0.03
Boiled potatoes	0.06
Cucumber	0.07
Cottage cheese	0.08
Full cream milk	0.09
Cabbage, boiled	0.10
Leg of lamb, cooked	0.10
Cauliflower	0.11
Roast chicken	0.11
Frozen peas	0.18
Red kidney beans, cooked	0.20
Wholemeal bread	0.20
Orange	0.24
Topside of beef, cooked	0.26
Banana	0.27
Brown rice, boiled	0.30
Grilled herring	0.30
Lamb's liver, fried	0.32
Baked beans	0.36
Corn flakes	0.40
Pear	0.50
Cheddar cheese	0.53
Carrots	0.56
Lettuce	0.57
Cox's apple	0.59
Grilled cod	0.59
Rice Krispies	0.60
Plums	0.61
Unsweetened orange juice	0.68
Leeks	0.78
Sweet corn, boiled	0.88
Brussels sprouts	0.90
Broccoli	1.10
Boiled egg	1.11
Tomato	1.22
Watercress	1.46
Parsley	1.70
Spinach, boiled	1.71
Olives	1.99
Butter	2.00
Onions, dried raw	2.69
Fried mushrooms	2.84
Avocado	3.20
Muesli	3.20
Walnuts	3.85
Peanut butter	4.99
Olive oil	5.10
Sweet potato, baked	5.96
Brazil nuts	7.18
Peanuts	10.09
Pine nuts	13.65
Rapeseed oil	18.40
Almonds	23.96
Hazelnuts	24.98
Sunflower oil	48.70

Calcium

Milligrams per 100g (3.5oz)

Cox's apple	4.00
Brown rice, boiled	4.00
Potatoes, boiled	5.00
Banana	6.00
Topside of beef, cooked	6.00
White pasta, boiled	7.00
Tomato	7.00
White spaghetti, boiled	7.00
Leg of lamb, cooked	8.00
Red bell peppers, raw	8.00
Roast chicken	9.00
Roast turkey	9.00
Avocado	11.0
Pear	11.0
Butter	15.0
Corn flakes	15.0
White rice, boiled	18.0
Grilled cod	22.0

Lentils, boiled	22.0
Baked salmon	29.0
Green bell peppers, raw	30.0
Young carrots	30.0
Grilled herring	33.0
Wholemeal flour	38.0
Turnips, baked	45.0
Orange	47.0
Baked beans	48.0
Wholemeal bread	54.0
Boiled egg	57.0
Peanuts	60.0
Cottage cheese	73.0
Soy beans, boiled	83.0
White bread	100.0
Full cream milk	115.0
Hovis	120.0
Muesli	120.0
Non-fat milk	120.0
2% reduced fat milk	120.0
Shrimps, boiled	150.0
Spinach, boiled	150.0
Brazil nuts	70.00
Yogurt, low-fat, plain	190.0
Soy flour	210.0
Almonds	240.0
White self-raising flour	450.0
Sardines	550.0
Sprats, fried	710.0
Cheddar cheese	720.0
Whitebait, fried	860.0

Chromium
Micrograms per 100g (3.5oz)

Fruit juices	47.0
Liver	55.0
Hard cheese	56.0
Beef	57.0
Brewer's yeast	117.0

Molasses	121.00
Egg yolk	183.00

Iron
Milligrams per 100g (3.5oz)

2% reduced fat milk	0.05
Non-fat milk	0.06
Full cream milk	0.06
Cottage cheese	0.10
Orange	0.10
Cox's apple	0.20
Pear	0.20
White rice	0.20
Banana	0.30
Cabbage, boiled	0.30
Cheddar cheese	0.30
Avocado	0.40
Grilled cod	0.40
Potatoes, boiled	0.40
Young carrots, boiled	0.40
Brown rice, boiled	0.50
Tomato	0.50
White pasta, boiled	0.50
Baked salmon	0.80
Roast chicken	0.80
Roast turkey	0.90
Grilled herring	1.00
Red bell peppers, raw	1.00
Boiled shrimps	1.10
Green bell peppers, raw	1.20
Baked beans	1.40
Cooked w/meal spaghetti	1.40
White bread	1.60
Spinach, boiled	1.70
Boiled egg	1.90
White self-raising flour	2.00
Brazil nuts	2.50
Peanuts	2.50
Leg of lamb, cooked	2.70

Wholemeal bread	2.70
Topside of beef, cooked	2.80
Almonds	3.00
Soy beans, boiled	3.00
Lentils, boiled	3.50
Hovis	3.70
Wholemeal flour	3.90
Muesli	5.60
Corn flakes	6.70
Rice Krispies	6.70
Soy flour	6.90

Magnesium
Milligrams per 100g (3.5oz)

Butter	2.00
Cox's apple	6.00
Turnip, baked	6.00
Young carrots	6.00
Tomato	7.00
Cottage cheese	9.00
Orange	10.00
Full cream milk	11.00
White rice, boiled	11.00
2% reduced fat milk	11.00
Non-fat milk	12.00
Boiled egg	12.00
Corn flakes	14.00
Potatoes, boiled	14.00
Red bell peppers, raw	14.00
White pasta, boiled	15.00
Cooked w/meal spaghetti	15.00
White self-raising flour	20.00
Green bell peppers, raw	24.00
Roast chicken	24.00
Topside of beef, cooked	24.00
White bread	24.00
Avocado	25.00
Cheddar cheese	25.00
Grilled cod	26.00

Roast turkey	27.0
Leg of lamb, cooked	28.0
Baked salmon	29.0
Baked beans	31.0
Spinach, boiled	31.0
Grilled herring	32.0
Banana	34.0
Lentils, boiled	34.0
Boiled shrimps	42.0
Wholemeal spaghetti	42.0
Brown rice, boiled	43.0
Hovis	56.0
Soy beans, boiled	63.0
Wholemeal bread	76.0
Muesli	85.0
Wholemeal flour	120.0
Peanuts	210.0
Soy flour	240.0
Almonds	270.0
Brazil nuts	410.0

Selenium
Micrograms per 100g (3.5oz)

Full cream milk	1.00
Non-fat milk	1.00
Baked beans	2.00
Corn flakes	2.00
Orange	2.00
Peanuts	3.00
Almonds	4.00
Cottage cheese	4.00
White rice	4.00
White self-raising flour	4.00
Soy beans, boiled	5.00
Boiled egg	11.00
Cheddar cheese	12.00
White bread	28.00
Wholemeal bread	35.00

Lentils, boiled	40.00
Wholemeal flour	53.00
Brazil nuts	1,900

Zinc
Milligrams per 100 g (3.5oz)

Butter	0.10
Pear	0.10
Orange	0.10
Red bell peppers, raw	0.10
Banana	0.20
Young carrots	0.20
Corn flakes	0.30
Potatoes, boiled	0.30
Avocado	0.40
Full cream milk	0.40
Non-fat milk	0.40
Green bell peppers, raw	0.40
2% reduced fat milk	0.40
Baked beans	0.50
Grilled cod	0.50
Grilled herring	0.50
White pasta	0.50
Tomatoes	0.50
Cottage cheese	0.60
Spinach, boiled	0.60
White bread	0.60
White self-raising flour	0.60
Brown rice	0.70
White rice	0.70
Soy beans, boiled	0.90
Cooked w/meal spaghetti	1.10
Boiled egg	1.30
Lentils, boiled	1.40
Roast chicken	1.50
Boiled shrimps	1.60
Wholemeal bread	1.80
Hovis	2.10

Cheddar cheese	2.30
Roast turkey	2.40
Muesli	2.50
Wholemeal flour	2.90
Almonds	3.20
Peanuts	3.50
Brazil nuts	4.20
Leg of lamb, cooked	5.30
Topside of beef, cooked	5.50

Essential Fatty Acids

Exact amounts of these fats are hard to quantify. Good sources for the two families of essential fatty acids are listed below.

Omega-6 Series Essential Fatty Acids

Sunflower oil
Rapeseed oil
Corn oil
Almonds
Walnuts
Brazil nuts
Sunflower seeds
Soy products including tofu

Omega-3 Series Essential Fatty Acids

Mackerel
Herring
Salmon
Trout
Avocado
Walnuts
Walnut oil
Rapeseed oil
Olive Oil

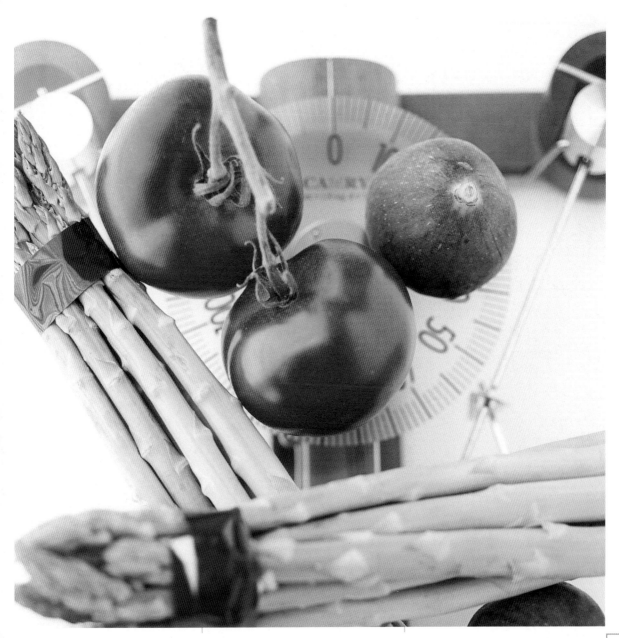

315

"I changed my diet... After a few weeks,
I had so much more energy
and my friends commented on how clear my skin looked."

Jean Cunningham

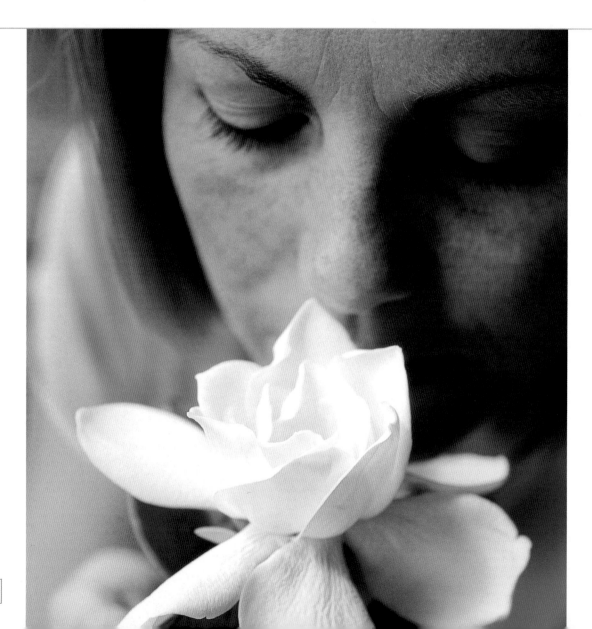

worksheets and diet diary

My Natural Menopause Plan

Summary of Recommendations

Diet

1. _____

2. _____

3. _____

4. _____

5. _____

6. _____

7. _____

8. _____

9. _____

10. _____

Supplements

1. _____

2. _____

3. _____

4. _____

5. _____

6. _____

Exercise and relaxation

1. _____

2. _____

3. _____

4. _____

Points to Remember

_____

_____

_____

_____

When you have finished compiling your program, pin it up somewhere visible, such as the outside of your refrigerator or on your kitchen bulletin board, so you can refer to it regularly.

My Self Assessment

Your Scores	Before	After
What is your body trying to tell you?	_____	_____
How strong are your bones?	_____	_____
Are you at risk of heart disease?	_____	_____
How's your libido?	_____	_____
How fit are you?	_____	_____
How do you see yourself?	_____	_____
How brain smart are you?	_____	_____
How stressed are you?	_____	_____
Is your diet good for you?	_____	_____
Are you a craver?	_____	_____
Is food the culprit?	_____	_____
Total Score	_____	_____

Deduct your After score from your Before score to get your:

Personal Balance Score (PBS)   _____

Possible nutritional deficiencies

Diet Diary (Complete on a Daily Basis for all Food and Drink Consumed)   Date_____

	Breakfast	Lunch	Dinner	Snacks	Exercise, symptoms, supplements
Day 1					
Day 2					
Day 3					
Day 4					
Day 5					
Day 6					
Day 7					

Diet Diary (Complete on a Daily Basis for all Food and Drink Consumed)   Date_____

	Breakfast	Lunch	Dinner	Snacks	Exercise, symptoms, supplements
Day 1					
Day 2					
Day 3					
Day 4					
Day 5					
Day 6					
Day 7					

© Copyright NHAS

Diet Diary (Complete on a Daily Basis for all Food and Drink Consumed)   Date_____

	Breakfast	Lunch	Dinner	Snacks	Exercise, symptoms, supplements
Day 1					
Day 2					
Day 3					
Day 4					
Day 5					
Day 6					
Day 7					

Diet Diary (Complete on a Daily Basis for all Food and Drink Consumed)   Date_____

	Breakfast	Lunch	Dinner	Snacks	Exercise, symptoms, supplements
Day 1					
Day 2					
Day 3					
Day 4					
Day 5					
Day 6					
Day 7					

Diet Diary (Complete on a Daily Basis for all Food and Drink Consumed)   Date_____

	Breakfast	Lunch	Dinner	Snacks	Exercise, symptoms, supplements
Day 1					
Day 2					
Day 3					
Day 4					
Day 5					
Day 6					
Day 7					

© Copyright NHAS

Diet Diary (Complete on a Daily Basis for all Food and Drink Consumed)   Date_____

	Breakfast	Lunch	Dinner	Snacks	Exercise, symptoms, supplements
Day 1					
Day 2					
Day 3					
Day 4					
Day 5					
Day 6					
Day 7					

Diet Diary (Complete on a Daily Basis for all Food and Drink Consumed)   Date_____

	Breakfast	Lunch	Dinner	Snacks	Exercise, symptoms, supplements
Day 1					
Day 2					
Day 3					
Day 4					
Day 5					
Day 6					
Day 7					

Diet Diary (Complete on a Daily Basis for all Food and Drink Consumed)   Date_____

	Breakfast	Lunch	Dinner	Snacks	Exercise, symptoms, supplements
Day 1					
Day 2					
Day 3					
Day 4					
Day 5					
Day 6					
Day 7					

Diet Diary (Complete on a Daily Basis for all Food and Drink Consumed)   Date_____

	Breakfast	Lunch	Dinner	Snacks	Exercise, symptoms, supplements
Day 1					
Day 2					
Day 3					
Day 4					
Day 5					
Day 6					
Day 7					

Diet Diary (Complete on a Daily Basis for all Food and Drink Consumed)   Date_____

	Breakfast	Lunch	Dinner	Snacks	Exercise, symptoms, supplements
Day 1					
Day 2					
Day 3					
Day 4					
Day 5					
Day 6					
Day 7					

Diet Diary (Complete on a Daily Basis for all Food and Drink Consumed)   Date_____

	Breakfast	Lunch	Dinner	Snacks	Exercise, symptoms, supplements
Day 1					
Day 2					
Day 3					
Day 4					
Day 5					
Day 6					
Day 7					

Diet Diary (Complete on a Daily Basis for all Food and Drink Consumed)   Date_____

	Breakfast	Lunch	Dinner	Snacks	Exercise, symptoms, supplements
Day 1					
Day 2					
Day 3					
Day 4					
Day 5					
Day 6					
Day 7					

Natural Health Advisory Service

Name _____

Grading of Symptoms

0	None	
1	Mild	present, but does not interfere with activities
2	Moderate	present and interferes with activities, but not disabling
3	Severe	disabling and unable to function

Date																		
Menses																		
Hot/cold flashes																		
Facial/body flashing																		
Night sweats																		
Palpitations																		
Panic attacks																		
Generalised aches & pains																		
Depression																		
Perspiration																		
Numbness/skin tingling																		
Headaches																		

Backache																			
Fatigue																			
Irritability																			
Nervousness																			
Insomnia																			
Giddiness/dizziness																			
Difficulty/frequent urination																			
Constipation																			
Itchy vagina																			
Dry vagina																			
Painful intercourse																			
Decreased sex drive																			
Loss of concentration																			
Confusion/loss of vitality																			
Water retention																			
Bloated abdomen																			
Weight (kg)																			
Sexual intercourse																			

Additional notes _____

335

Menopause Symptomatology Diary

Natural Health Advisory Service

Name _____

Grading of Symptoms

0	None	
1	Mild	present, but does not interfere with activities
2	Moderate	present and interferes with activities, but not disabling
3	Severe	disabling and unable to function

Date																			
Menses																			
Hot/cold flashes																			
Facial/body flashing																			
Night sweats																			
Palpitations																			
Panic attacks																			
Generalised aches & pains																			
Depression																			
Perspiration																			
Numbness/skin tingling																			
Headaches																			

Backache																			
Fatigue																			
Irritability																			
Nervousness																			
Insomnia																			
Giddiness/dizziness																			
Difficulty/frequent urination																			
Constipation																			
Itchy vagina																			
Dry vagina																			
Painful intercourse																			
Decreased sex drive																			
Loss of concentration																			
Confusion/loss of vitality																			
Water retention																			
Bloated abdomen																			
Weight (kg)																			
Sexual intercourse																			

Additional notes _____

337

Menopause Symptomatology Diary

Natural Health Advisory Service

Name _____

Grading of Symptoms

0	None	
1	Mild	present, but does not interfere with activities
2	Moderate	present and interferes with activities, but not disabling
3	Severe	disabling and unable to function

Date																			
Menses																			
Hot/cold flashes																			
Facial/body flashing																			
Night sweats																			
Palpitations																			
Panic attacks																			
Generalised aches & pains																			
Depression																			
Perspiration																			
Numbness/skin tingling																			
Headaches																			

Backache																		
Fatigue																		
Irritability																		
Nervousness																		
Insomnia																		
Giddiness/dizziness																		
Difficulty/frequent urination																		
Constipation																		
Itchy vagina																		
Dry vagina																		
Painful intercourse																		
Decreased sex drive																		
Loss of concentration																		
Confusion/loss of vitality																		
Water retention																		
Bloated abdomen																		
Weight (kg)																		
Sexual intercourse																		

Additional notes _____

339

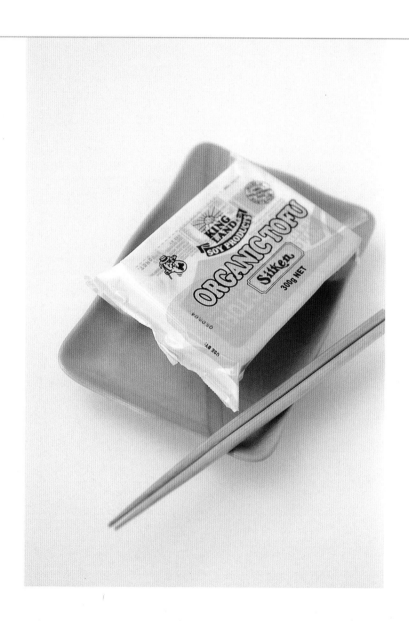

Phytoestrogen-rich Food in the USA
Spelling of soy may be varied to soya where products are imported

Soy-Containing Foods Meat Substitutes & Entrees

Amy's Tofu Vegetable Lasagna
Amy's Macaroni and Soy Cheese
Amy's Tofu Scramble with Hash Browns and Vegetables
Amy's Tofu Rancheros
Lightlife Smart Bacon
Lightlife Smart BBQ Shredded Veggie Protein in BBQ Sauce
Lightlife Smart Menu, Orange Sesame Chick'n or Garlic Teriyaki Chick'n
Midland Harvest Mixes, Taco, Burger or Chili
Midland Harvest Crumbles
Midland Harvest Chik'n for Recipes
Midland Harvest Breaded Chicken-Style Patty or Nuggets
Midland Harvest Chargrilled Veggie Burger
Midland Harvest Vegan Burger
Midland Harvest Savory Breakfast Patty or Links
Midland Harvest Savory Meatball
Boca Meatless Burgers (6 varieties)*
Boca Meatless Sausages, Italian Sausage, Smoked Sausage or Bratwurst
Boca Meatless Breakfast, Breakfast Patties or Links
Boca Meatless Chik'n Patties, Original or Spicy*
Boca Meatless Chik'n Nuggets, Original*
Boca Meatless Rising Crust Pizza, Supreme or Pepperoni*
Boca Meatless Lasagna
Boca Meatless Chili
Boca Meatless Burger w/Organic Soy (6 varieties)
Boca Meatless Burgers (5 Varieties)
Boca Meatless Sausages w/No Artificial Preservatives or Flavors, Italian Sausage or Bratwurst
Boca Meatless Breakfast w/Organic Soy, Breakfast Patties or Links
Boca Meatless Chik'n Wings w/No Artificial Preservatives or Flavors, Hot & Spicy

Gardenburger BBQ Riblets
Gardenburger Veggie Medley Veggie Burgers
Health Valley Chunky Chili (7 varieties)
Health is Wealth Spinach Egg Rolls
Health is Wealth Pizza Munchees
Veggie Patch Nuggets, Broccoli or Spinach
Veggie Patch Meatless Meatballs
Veggie Patch Meatless Garlic Portabella Burgers
Veggie Patch Meatless Gourmet Sausage (5 varieties)
Franklin Farms Fresh Veggiburger, Original Recipe or Portabella
Yves Veggie Cuisine, Burgers (4 varieties)
Yves Veggie Cuisine, Canadian Veggie Bacon
Yves Veggie Cuisine, Veggie Breakfast Patties or Links
Yves Veggie Cuisine, Veggie Pizza, Pepperoni
Yves Veggie Cuisine, Veggie Slices, Ham, Turkey, Bologna or Salami
Yves Veggie Cuisine, Veggie Meatballs
Yves Veggie Cuisine, Veggie Ground Round, Original or Mexican
Yves Veggie Cuisine, Dogs, Veggie, Hot 'n' Spicy, Jumbo or Tofu
Yves Veggie Cuisine, Veggie Lasagna
Yves Veggie Cuisine, Veggie Chili
Yves Veggie Cuisine, Classic Mac 'n' Soy Cheese
Yves Veggie Cuisine, Veggie Penne
Yves Veggie Cuisine, Santa Fe Veggie Beef
Yves Veggie Cuisine, Thai Lemongrass Veggie Chick'n
Yves Meatless Skewers BBQ Beef or Lemon Herb Chicken
Morning Star Farms Veggie Bites, Spinach Artichoke or Broccoli Cheddar
MorningStar Farms Veggie Burgers (9 varieties)*
MorningStar Farms Chik, Buffalo Wings
MorningStar Farms Chik, Chik'n Nuggets
Morning Star Farms Chicken Strips
MorningStar Farms Chik, Patties Breaded, Veggie or Parmesan Ranch
MorningStar Farms Chik, Original Chik'n Tenders
MorningStar Farms Breakfast (6 varieties)

MorningStar Farms Meal Starters, Crumbles, Grillers Recipe or Sausage Style
MorningStar Farms Meal Starters, Steak or Chik'n Strips
MorningStar Farms Dogs, America's Original, Corn or Mini
MorningStar Farms Snacks, Veggie Bites Spinach Artichoke or Broccoli Cheddar
MorningStar Farms w/Organic Soy, Okara or Veggie Breakfast Patties
MorningStar Farms w/Organic Soy, Roasted Herb Chik'n
Worthington Chili
Worthington meat substitute, Choplets or Tender Round meatballs
Worthington meat substitute, Skallops or Veja-Links
Worthington Loma Linda Linketts protein links, Little Links, Super-Links
Worthington Diced Chik
Worthington FriChik chicken substitute
Worthington Loma Linda Big Franks, Dinner Cuts
Worthington Loma Linda, Low Fat Big Franks, Tender Bits
Worthington Loma Linda patties, Vege-Burger or Redi-Burger
Worthington Multi-Grain Cutlets, Prime Stakes
Worthington Saucettes
Worthington Turkee Slices
Worthington Vegetarian Burger
Tofurky Deli Slices, Italian Deli, Cranberry and Stuffing, Hickory Smoked, Oven Roasted
Tofurky Kielbasa, Italian Sausage, Beer Brats
Tofutti Pizza Pizzaz
Tofutti Mintz's Blintzes
Tofutti Cheese Pillow, Blueberry, Apple or Cherry
House Tofu Shirataki, Fettuccine Shape or Noodle Shaped
Marjon Tofu, Firm, Grilled, Crumbles
Marjon Tofu Grills, Hickory Sizzler, Zesty Herb, and Mesquite Pepper Rub
Heartland Fields All-Natural Meals (4 varieties)
White Wave Seitan, Traditional, Stir Fry, Chicken Style or Chicken Style Meat of Wheat

Soymilk

WestSoy Soymilk Plus, Plain or Vanilla
WestSoy Low Fat Soymilk, Plain or Vanilla
WestSoy Soymilk Lite, Plain or Vanilla
WestSoy Non Fat Soymilk, Plain or Vanilla
WestSoy Soymilk, Organic Original
WestSoy Unsweetened Soymilk (4 flavors)
West Soy Soy Slender Soymilk (4 flavors)
Silk Creamer, Original, French Vanilla or Hazelnut
Silk Soymilk, Refrigerated, Plain, Vanilla, or Chocolate
Silk Soymilk Light, Refrigerated, Plain, Vanilla or Chocolate
Silk Soymilk, Refrigerated (6 varieties)
8th Continent Soymilk, Original, Vanilla or Chocolate
8th Continent Soymilk, Light, Original, Vanilla or Chocolate
8th Continent Soymilk, Fat Free, Original or Vanilla
Edensoy Soymilk, Organic (9 varieties)
VitaSoy Soymilk (8 varieties)
VitaSoy Soymilk, Complete Original or Vanilla
ZenSoy Soymilk, Plain, Vanilla, Chocolate or Cappuccino

Soy Drinks, Shakes & Powders

Revival Chocolate Daydream Shake
Revival Vanilla Pleasure Shake
Revival Strawberry Smile Shake
Revival Cappuccino Comfort Shake
Revival Just Peachy Shake
Revival Banana Blessings Shake
Revival Strawberry Banana Bliss Shake
Revival Blueberry Blush
Revival Plain/Organic Soy Shake
Genisoy MLO Powder, Super High Protein or Vegetable Protein
Genisoy Ultra XT Protein Shake Powder, Natural, Vanilla or Chocolate
Genisoy Protein Shake Powder, Natural, Vanilla, Strawberry Banana or Chocolate
WestSoy Soy Shake, Vanilla or Chocolate
Silk Live Smoothie, Blueberry, Mango, Peach, Raspberry or

Strawberry
Whole Soy & Co. Organic Soy Smoothie, Peach, Strawberry,
Raspberry or Apricot/Mango
8th Continent Refreshers, Strawberry Banana or Orange
Pineapple Banana
VitaSoy Light Soy Drink, Vanilla or Chocolate
VitaSoy Holly Nog or Peppermint Chocolate
VitaSoy Nutrifull Meal Replacement, Strawberry, Mixed
Berry or Mango Peach
Silk Soymilk (8 varieties)
Silk Coffee
Silk Mocha
8th Continent Soymilk (6 flavors)
Silk Live! Smoothie, Strawberry, Peach, Raspberry or
Mango
Soy Dream Vanilla Classic Soymilk (4 varieties)
Eden Soy Organic Soymilk (7 varieties)
Eden Blend Rice and Soy Beverage
Genisoy Soy Protein Shake, Chocolate or Vanilla
Naturade Total Soy Meal Replacement (3 flavors)

Soy Bars

Luna Whole Natural Bars For Women (8 varieties)
Luna Sunrise Yogurt Bar, Blueberry or Strawberry Cream
Clif Bar (6 flavors)
Power Bar Pria Nutrition Bars (4 flavors)
Power Bar Pria Grain Essentials Nutrition Bar (3 flavors)
Revival Smart-Carb Chocolate Peanut Paradise
Revival Smart-Carb Chocolate Raspberry Zing
Revival Smart-Carb Autumn Apple Frost
Revival Peanut Chocolate Buddy
Revival Peanut Pal
Revival Chocolate Temptation
Revival Apple Cinnamon Celebration
Revival Marshmallow Krunch
Dr. Soy Protein Bar (6 flavors)
Genisoy Ultra Bar (4 flavors)
Genisoy Cookies & Cream

Genisoy Chocolate Mint
Genisoy Creamy Peanut Yogurt
Genisoy Fudge, Chunky Peanut Butter or Café Mocha
Fudge
Genisoy Chocolate Fudge Brownie
Genisoy Natural Choice (4 varieties)
Genisoy Low Carb Crunch (4 varieties)
Genisoy MLO Xtreme Bar (4 varieties)
Genisoy MLO Bio Protein Bar (4 varieties)
Zoe's Bars (4 varieties)

Soy Snacks

Revival Lightly Salted Sunshine Soy Protein Chips
Revival Oh My! Apple Pie Soy Protein Chips
Revival BBQ Bliss Soy Protein Chips
Revival Sour Cream N' Onion Dream Soy Protein Chips
Revival Roasted Garlic & Herbs Goodness
Soy Protein Chips
Revival Salsa Sass Soy Protein Chips
Revival Jalapeno N' Cheddar Cha Cha Soy Protein Chips
Revival Rev-It-Up Ranch Soy Protein Chips
Revival Sea Salt & Vinegar Voyage Soy Protein Chips
Revival Honey Mustard Heaven Soy Protein Chips
Revival Naturally Nice Soy Protein Chips
Revival Soynuts (8 varieties)
Amport Foods Lightly Salted Soy Nuts
Amport Foods Honey Roasted Soy Nuts
Dr. Soy Trail Mix, California Blend Soy or Tropical Blend
Dr. Soy Soy Nuts, Original, Barbecue, Chocolate or Ranch
Genisoy Potato Soy Crisps (4 flavors)
Genisoy Soy Crisps (8 flavors)
Genisoy Soytato Chips, Lightly Salted, Sour Cream & Onion
or Barbeque
Genisoy Soy Nuts (5 flavors)
Genisoy Trail Mix (3 flavors)
Hain PureSnax Soy Munchies (3 flavors)
Robert's American Gourmet Soy Crisps (3 flavors)

Soy Pasta

Revival Soy Pasta, Thin Spaghetti
Revival Soy Pasta, Angel Hair
Revival Soy Pasta, Penne
Revival Soy Pasta, Rotini
Midland Harvest, Angel Hair, Elbow Macaroni, Lasagna, Penne, Rigate, Rotini or Spaghetti
Azumaya Pasta, Noodles, Thin Cut or Wide
Azumaya Pasta, Wrappers, Large Square, Square or Round

Soups

Health Valley Soup, Fat Free Pasta Parmesan
Westbrae Natural, Miso (10 varieties)
Eden Foods, Miso, Organic (4 varieties)

Soy Coffee

Revival Breakfast In Bed Blend
Revival Original Roast Romance
Revival Dark Roast Diva
Revival French Vanilla Flirt
Revival Hazelnut Hugs & Kisses
Revival Will You Mocha Me
Soyfee (6 varieties)

Yogurts

Silk Yogurt (8 flavors)
Whole Soy & Co. Soy Yogurt (12 flavors)
Whole Soy & Co. Soy Frozen Yogurt (9 flavors)

Tempeh and Tofu

White Wave Tempeh, Original Soy, Five Grain or Soy Rice
TofuTown Tofu Tenders (4 varieties)
White Wave Baked Tofu (5 varieties)
White Wave Tofu, Extra Firm Style
White Wave Tofu, Organic Extra Firm, Firm or Soft Style
White Wave Tofu, Reduced Fat
Toby's Tofu Pate (5 varieties)
FarmSoy Tofu, Firm or Extra Firm Style
Azumaya Tofu, Firm, Silken, Extra Firm

Azumaya Tofu, Lite Extra Firm or Silken
Azumaya Tofu, Super Firm Cubed, Oriental Spice or Zesty Garlic & Onion
Mori-Nu Silken Tofu, Extra Firm, Soft, Extra Firm Lite
Organic Nasoya Tofu, Firm, Extra Firm, Lite Firm, Soft, Cubed, Silken

Cereals

Health Valley, Slender, Raisin Soy Flakes or Heart Wise
Zoe's O's Cereal, Natural, Honey or Cinnamon
Zoe's Granola Cereal, Cranberries Currant, Honey Almond or Cinnamon Raisin
Breadshop's Granola, Blueberry 'n Cream or Strawberry 'n Cream
Kashi Go Lean High Protein and High Fiber Cereal
Nutritious Living Hi-Lo 100% Natural Original Flavor
Nature's Path Organic Optimum Slim Cereal
Nature's Path Organic Optimum Zen Cranberry-Ginger

Spreads and Breads

All Natural Soy Wonder Crunchy, Peanut Butter flavor
French Meadow Bakery Women's Loaf
Galaxy Nutritional Foods Veggie Butter Alternative
Nasoya All Natural Mayonnaise

Cheese Substitutes

Galaxy Nutritional Foods Veggie Shreds, Cheddar or Mozzarella
Galaxy Nutritional Foods Veggie Pasteurized Cheese Food Alternative
Galaxy Nutritional Foods Veggie Slices (5 varieties)
Tofutti Better Than Cream Cheese (6 flavors)
Tofutti Soy-Cheese Slices, Mozzarella, American or Roasted Garlic

Desserts

Joelle's Choice Pudding, Vanilla or Chocolate
Tofutti Non-Dairy Frozen Dessert (18 flavors)
Tofutti Cuties (13 flavors)

Tofutti Dessert Bars (8 flavors)
Tofutti Tofiggy Fig Bars
Tofutti Cookies (3 varieties)
Soy Delicious Purely Decadent Non-Dairy
Frozen Dessert (15 flavors)
Soy Delicious Purely Decadent Non-Dairy Frozen Stickbars,
Purely or Almond Vanilla
Soy Delicious Purely Decadent Non-Dairy Frozen Coated
Sandwich, Mocha or Vanilla Mania
So Delicious Dairy Free Frozen Bars (3 flavors)
Organic So Delicious Non-Dairy Frozen
Dessert Quarts (12 flavors)
Organic So Delicious Non-Dairy Frozen
Dessert Novelties (9 varieties)
Organic So Delicious Non-Dairy Frozen Dessert,
Li'l Buddies (4 flavors)
So Delicious Dairy Free, Sugar Free Novelty,
Vanilla or Fudge Bar
It's Soy Delicious Fruit Sweetened Non-Dairy Frozen
Dessert Pints (14 flavors)
ZenSoy Pudding, Chocolate, Vanilla, Banana or Chocolate/
Vanilla Swirl

Baking Products

Arrowhead Mills Organic Soy flour
Cascadian Farms Frozen Edamame
Sunrich Natural Edamame
Seapoint Farms Edamame Soybean in Pod
Seapoint Farms Edamame Shelled Soybean
Natural Products Roasted Full Fat Soy Flour
Natural Products Roasted Full Fat Soy Meal
Natural Products Roasted Full Fat Soy Grits
Natural Products Low Fat Soy Flour

Other Products

Westbrae Natural Organic Soy Beans
Bright Beginnings Soy Pediatric Drink
I.M. Healthy SoyNut Butter (7 varieties)Eden Foods, Black
Soybeans, Organic

Phytoestrogen-rich Food in Canada

Drinks

So Good Fortified Soy Beverage (5 varieties and flavors)
Provamel chocolate soy drink
Sensational Soy with Omega 3 Creamy, Classic Vanilla and
Smooth Chocolate

Spreads and breads

Vogel's brown soya bread
Galaxy Veggie Butter flavor Spread
Stonemill Soy Source 3 Gran Bread
President's Choice Blue Menu Multi Grain Flax Loaf
President's Choice Blue Menu Raisin Bran Flax Muffins
President's Choice Blue Menu Whole Wheat Soy LoafI.M.
Healthy SoyNut Butter (7 varieties)

Cheese substitutes

Toffiti cream-cheese-style with original, herbs and chives
and garlic and herbs
Toffiti mozzarella-style slices

Meat substitutes

Unisoya Soya & Vegetable Wieners
Yves Spicy Italian Sausage
Yves The Good Veggie Burger
Yves Ground Round

Desserts

Tofutti organic soya dessert, chocolate or mango/
passionfruit
Pete's Tofu Deserts (assorted flavors)
So Yummi Soy Mousse (assorted flavors)
Life Stream Soy Plus Optimum Power Waffles,
Flax, Soy, Blueberry

Cereals and nuts

CanMar golden roasted milled flax seed with
real blueberries

CanMar golden roasted milled flax seed with real apples
CanMar golden roasted milled flax seed, ready to eat
CanMar whole roasted flax seeds
Natural Harvest soya bran
Vogels soya and linseed cereal
Natures Path organic power cereal with flaxseed, soy, blueberry
Bob's Red Mill Right Stuff 6 Grain Hot Cereal with Flax seed, Organic

Cooking

Bob's Red Mill Soy Flour, (including low fat)
Bob's Red Mill Soy Beans
Bob's Red Mill Flax Seed Meal (Golden)
Yves canned Soy Beans
Bragg's All purpose Seasoning, Liquid Soy

Snacks

Inari Dry Soy Beans
Skeet and Ikes Soy Nuts
Meat Substitutes & Entrees
*Varieties available with a choice of Soy, Organic Soy or Additive Free
Boca Meatless Burgers (6 varieties)*
Boca Meatless Sausages (3 varieties)*
Boca Meatless Breakfast, Breakfast Patties or Links*
Boca Meatless Chik'n Patties, Original or Spicy*
Boca Meatless Chik'n Nuggets, Original*
Boca Meatless Ground Burger*
Boca Meatless Rising Crust Pizza, Supreme, Pepperoni and Tomato*
Boca Meatless Lasagna
Boca Meatless Chili
Boca Meatless Chik'n Wings w/No Artificial Preservatives or Flavors, Hot & Spicy
Health Valley Chunky Chili, Spicy Vegetarian, Black Bean
Yves Veggie Cuisine, Burgers (6 varieties)
Yves Veggie Cuisine, Canadian Veggie Bacon
Yves Veggie Cuisine, Veggie Breakfast Patties or Links

Yves Veggie Cuisine, Veggie Pizza, Pepperoni
Yves Veggie Cuisine, Veggie Slices, Ham, Turkey, Bologna or Salami
Yves Veggie Cuisine, Veggie Cajun Chicken or Ground Chicken
Yves Veggie Cuisine, Veggie Roast Beef
Yves Veggie Cuisine, Veggie Meatballs
Yves Veggie Cuisine, Veggie Ground Round, Original or Mexican
Yves Veggie Cuisine, Veggie Dogs, Chili Dogs or Tofu Dogs
Yves Veggie Cuisine, Spicy Veggie Sausage, Italian or Bavarian
Yves Veggie Cuisine, Veggie Lasagna
Yves Veggie Cuisine, Veggie Chili
Yves Veggie Cuisine, Classic Mac 'n' Soy Cheese
Yves Veggie Cuisine, Veggie Penne
Yves Veggie Cuisine, Santa Fe Veggie Beef
Yves Veggie Cuisine, Thai Lemongrass Veggie Chick'n
Yves Veggie Cuisine, Veggie Tenders, Chicken or Beef
MorningStar Farms Veggie Burgers* (9 varieties)
MorningStar Farms Chik, Buffalo Wings
MorningStar Farms Chik, Chik'n Nuggets
MorningStar Farms Chik, Patties, Breaded Veggie or Parmesan Ranch
MorningStar Farms Chik, Original Chik'n Tenders
MorningStar Farms Breakfast, Better'n Eggs
MorningStar Farms Breakfast, Veggie Breakfast Bacon, Links, Scramblers or Patties*
MorningStar Farms Breakfast, Breakfast Sandwich with Cheese
MorningStar Farms Meal Starters (4 varieties)
MorningStar Farms Dogs, America's Original or Corn Dogs Veggie Dog
MorningStar Farms Snacks, Veggie Bites Spinach Artichoke or Broccoli Cheddar
MorningStar Farms w/Organic Soy, Roasted Herb Chik'n
Tofutti Pizza Pizzaz
Tofutti Mintz's Blintzes
Tofutti Cheese Pillow, Blueberry, Apple or Cherry

365 Organic Veggie Burger, Vegan or Classic
Money's Garden Burger (4 varieties)
President's Choice Blue Menu Soy Burgers
President's Choice Blue Menu Soy Deli slices
President's Choice Blue Menu Hot Dogs
President's Choice blue Menu Ground Soy
Sol Cuisine T-Ribz
Sol Cuisine Vegetable Burger
Sol Cuisine Falafel
Tofurky Tofu Sausage, Beer, Italian or Kielbasa
Tofurky Slices, Italian Deli, Hickory Smoked or Oven
Roasted
Zoglo's Crispy Meatless Cutlets
Zoglo's Meatless Burgers, Wieners, Kebabs or Nuggets
Zoglo's Spinach Cutlets
Zoglo's Patties, Broccoli or Vegetable
Soya Nova Westcoast Smoked Tofu
So Soya Ground Veggie Burger
So Soya Veggie Chick'n Strips
So Soya Instant Meals, Oriental Teriyaki or Thai
So Soya Combos, Teriyaki, Lemon Garlic Herb, Jamaican
Jerk or Honey Dijon

Soymilk

President's Choice Blue Menu Fortified Soy Beverages
Sensational Soy with Omega 3 (3 flavors)
Silk Creamer, Original, French Vanilla, Hazelnut
Silk Soymilk, Refrigerated, (4 flavors)
Silk Soymilk Light, Refrigerated (3 flavors)
Silk Soymilk, Refrigerated, Unsweetened
Silk Soymilk, Refrigerated, Enhanced
Silk Soymilk, Refrigerated (4 flavors)
So Good Fortified Soy Beverage (9 varieties and flavors)
SoySolutions Original, Almond, Chocolate or Vanilla
SoySolutionsRice Vanilla or Original
Edensoy Soymilk, Organic, Original, Carob,
Chocolate or Vanilla
Edensoy Soymilk, Organic Extra Original or Vanilla
Edensoy Soymilk, Organic Light Original or Vanilla

Edensoy Soymilk, Organic Unsweetened
VitaSoy Soymilk, Classic Original
VitaSoy Soymilk, Creamy Original
VitaSoy Soymilk, Vanilla, Gree Tea or Rich Chocolate
VitaSoy Soymilk, Original, Light or Unsweetened
VitaSoy Soymilk, Complete Original or Vanilla
365 Organic Soymilk, Original, Vanilla or Chocolate
Soy Dream Soymilk, Original or Vanilla

Soy Drinks, Shakes & Powders

Genisoy MLO Powder, Super High Protein or
Vegetable Protein
Genisoy Ultra XT Protein Shake Powder, Vanilla,
Chocolate or Natural
Genisoy Protein Shake Powder, Vanilla, Strawberry Banana,
Natural or Chocolate
WestSoy Soy Shake, Vanilla or Chocolate
Sensational Soy Omega 3 Smoothie Strawberry,
Orange or Banana
Sensational Soy Omega 3 Smoothie Orange,
Peach or Mango
Silk Live Smoothie, Blueberry, Mango, Peach,
Raspberry or Strawberry
VitaSoy Light Soy Drink, Vanilla or Chocolate
VitaSoy Holly Nog or Peppermint Chocolate
VitaSoy Nutrifull Meal Replacement, Strawberry, Mixed
Berry or Mango Peach
Yü Soy Beverage, Original, Almond Multigrain
or Vanilla Multigrain
Natura Soy Beverage, Original (6 varieties or flavors)
So Nice Soy Beverage, Natural (5 flavors)
InterACTIVE Nutrition SoyOne Protein Drink for
Women (3 flavors)
El Peto Soya Milk Powder

Soy Bars

Genisoy Ultra Bar (4 varieties)
Genisoy Cookies & Cream
Genisoy Chocolate Mint

Genisoy Creamy Peanut Yogurt
Genisoy Chunky Peanut Butter Fudge
Genisoy Chocolate Fudge Brownie
Genisoy Café Mocha Fudge
Genisoy Natural Choice (4 flavors)
Genisoy Low Carb Crunch (4 flavors)
Genisoy MLO Xtreme Bar (4 flavors)
Genisoy MLO Bio Protein Bar (4 flavors)
Zoe's Bars, Chocolate Peanut Butter, Chocolate, Apple
Clif Bar, Assorted Flavors
Clif Luna Bar, Assorted Flavors
Zone Perfect, Assorted Flavors
Nature's Path Optimum Energy Bar, Blueberry, Flax and Soy
Nature's Path Optimum Energy Bar, Cranberry,
Ginger and Soy

Soy Pasta

Midland Harvest, Angel Hair, Spaghetti, Lasagna, Penne,
Rotini or Elbow Macaroni
Azumaya Pasta, Noodles, Thin Cut or Wide Cut
Azumaya Pasta, Large Square Wrappers
Azumaya Pasta, Wrappers, Square or Round
Nutrition Kitchen, Angelhair, Whole Green, Golden or
Black Soybean

Soups

Health Valley Soup, Fat Free Pasta Parmesan
Westbrae Natural, Miso (10 varieties)

Eden Foods, Miso, Organic (4 varieties) Soy Snacks
Genisoy Potato Soy Crisp (4 varieties)
Genisoy Soy Crisps (8 varieties)
Genisoy Soytato Chips (3 varieties)
Genisoy Soy Nuts (5 varieties)
Genisoy Trail Mix (3 varieties)
Hain PureSnax Soy Munchies, White Cheddar,
Caramel or Ranch
Robert's American Gourmet Soy Crisps (3 varieties)

Skeet and Ikes Soy Nuts
Simply by Nature Soy Nuts, Roasted and Salted
Old Oakville Potato Soya Krisps, Sour Cream and Onion
or Honey BBQ
Old Oakville Corn Soya Tortillas, Ranch or Salsa Sour Cream
Pete's Tofu 2 Go Snackables Sesamee (4 varieties)
So Soya Crunchers, Sea Salted or Unsalted

Yogurts

Silk Yogurt (8 flavors)
YoSo Soy Yogurt, Assorted Flavors

Tempeh and Tofu

Noble Bean Tempeh, (4 varieties)
Azumaya Tofu, Firm, Extra Firm, Silken, Lite and Flavored
Mori-nu Tofu, Silken Soft, Firm, Extra Firm and Lite and
Flavored
Sol Cuisine Tofu, Firm
Pete's Tofu, Super Firm and Flavored
President' Choice Blue Menu Low Fat Tofu, Silken, Firm and
Flavored
Sunrise Tofu, Soft, Medium and Extra Firm
Unisoy Tofu (4 varieties)
Unisoy Organic (6 varieties)
365 Organic Tofu, Firm, Extra Firm
La Soyarie Tofu, Extra Firm or Herb

Cereals

Health Valley, Slender, Raisin Soy Flakes or Heartwise
Zoe's O's Cereal, Honey, Natural or Cinnamon
Zoe's Granola Cereal, Cranberries Currant, Honey Almond
or Cinnamon Raisin
Nature's Path Cereal, Soy Plus Granola
Nature's Path Optimum Power Cereal, Flax, Soy, Blueberry
Nature's Path Optimum Rebound Cereal (5 varieties)
Nutritious Living Hi-Lo Cereal, Original or Strawberry
Nutritious Living Dr. Sears Zone Cereal, Honey Almond
President's Choice Blue Menu Soy Crunch

Multi Grain Cereal
President's Choice Blue Menu Granola Cereal Original,
Raisin & Almond, Natural Wheat Bran
Kashi Go Lean Cereal
Kashi Go Lean Crunch Cereal

Cheese Substitutes
Tofutti Better Than Cream Cheese (6 falvors)
Tofutti Soy-Cheese Slices, Mozzarella, American
or Roasted Garlic
Galaxy Vegan Singles, American, Italian
Galaxy Blocks, Cheddar Flavour, Mozzarella Flavour
Sunergia Soya Feta, Tomato Garlic, Italian Herb,
Mediterranean or Lemon Oregano
Vegan Gourmet Cheese Alternatives, Soya Nacho Flavour
Yves the Good Slice Cheddar, Mozarella, Swiss

Desserts
Joelle's Choice Pudding, Chocolate or Vanilla
President's Choice Blue Menu Silken Tofu
Dessert Almond Flavor
So Good Non Dairy Non Dairy Frozen Dessert (5 flavors)
So Good Non Dairy Frozen Cones Chocolate or Vanilla
Tofutti Non-Dairy Frozen Dessert (7 flavors)
Tofutti Non-Dairy Frozen Dessert, Low Fat (3 flavors)
Tofutti Non-Dairy Frozen Dessert, No Sugar Added,
Strawberry or Chocolate
Tofutti Non-Dairy Frozen Dessert, Super Soy Supreme
(3 flavors)
Tofutti Non-Dairy Frozen Dessert, Cheesecake Supreme
(3 flavors)
Tofutti Cuties (13 flavors)
Tofutti Dessert Bars (8 varieties)
Tofutti Tofiggy Fig Bars
Tofutti Cookies (3 varieties)
Soy Delicious Purely Decadent Non-Dairy Frozen Dessert
(15 flavors)
Soy Delicious Purely Decadent Non-Dairy Frozen Stickbars,

Purely or Almond Vanilla
Soy Delicious Purely Decadent Non-Dairy Frozen Coated
Sandwich (2 flavors)
So Delicious Dairy Free Frozen Bars (3 flavors)
Organic So Delicious Non-Dairy Frozen Dessert Quarts
(12 flavors)
Organic So Delicious Non-Dairy Frozen Dessert Novelties
(9 varieties)
Organic So Delicious Non-Dairy Frozen Dessert, Li'l
Buddies (4 flavors)
So Delicious Dairy Free, Sugar Free Novelty, Fudge or
Vanilla Bar
It's Soy Delicious Fruit Sweetened Non-Dairy Frozen
Dessert Pints (14 flavors)
SoYummi Soy Mousse, Dark Chocolate, Bavarian Cream or
Black Cherry
Soy Dream Non-Dairy Frozen Dessert, Assorted Flavors
Double Rainbow Soy Cream, Assorted Flavors
Pete's Tofu Desserts (4 flavors)

Baking Products
Purely Bulk Fat Free Soy Flour
Bob's Red Mill Soy Flour
Bob's Red Mill Soy Grits (defatted)
El Peto Soya Flour, Low Fat

Other Products
Westbrae Natural Organic Soy Beans
Bright Beginnings Soy Pediatric Drink
Tofutti Sour Supreme, Plain or Guacamole
Eden Foods, Black Soybeans, Organic
I.M. Healthy SoyNut Butter (7 varieities)
Stonemill Soy Source 3 Grain Bread
Inari Dry Soy Beans
Yves Canned Soy Beans
Lifestream SoyPlus Optimum Power Waffles, Flax, Soy,
Blueberry
Bragg's All Purpose Seasoning, Liquid Soy

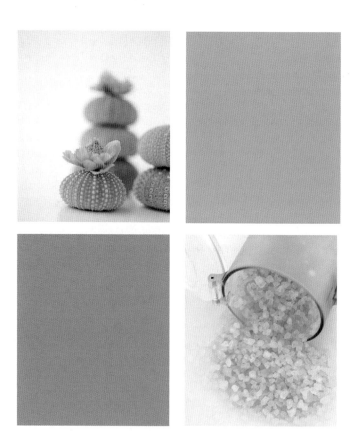

references

Standard References

1. American Medical Association. *Essential Guide to Menopause*. New York: Pocket Books, 2004.

2. Baik HW, Russell RM. Vitamin B12 deficiency in the elderly. *Annual Review of Nutrition*. 1999; 19:357-77

3. Bruinsma (Morris) K, Taren DL. Chocolate; food or drug? *J Ame Diet Assoc*. 1999; 99:1249-1256

4. Berg G, Hammar M (eds). *The modern management of the menopause*. New York; London: Parthenon Publishing, 1994.

5. Dennerstein L, Wood C, Westmore A. *Hysterectomy: new options and advances*, 2nd edn. Melbourne; Oxford: Oxford University Press, 1995.

6. Pizzorno JE, Murray MT (eds). *Textbook of natural medicine*. Edinburgh: Churchill Livingstone, 1999.

7. Souhami RL, Moxham J (eds). *Textbook of medicine,* 4th edn. Edinburgh: Churchill Livingstone, 2002.

8. Stewart M. *Cruising through the menopause.* London: Vermilion, 2000.

9. Stewart M, Stewart A. *The natural health bible: an A-Z guide to drug-free health.* Sydney: New Holland, 2002.

10. Stewart M. *The phyto factor.* London: Vermilion, 2000.

11. Werbach MR. *Textbook of Nutritional Medicine*. California: Third Line Press, 1999.

Menopause

12. Anderson GL, Limacher M, Assaf AR, *et al*. Effects of conjugated equine estrogen in postmenopausal women with hysterectomy: the Women's Health Initiative randomised controlled trial. *JAMA* 2004; **291**(14): 1701-12.

13. Chung TK, Yip SK, Lam P, Chang AM, Haines CJ. A randomized, double-blind, placebo-controlled,

14. Hale GE, Hughes CL, Robboy SJ, Agarwal SK, Bievre M. A double-blind randomized study on the effects of red clover isoflavones on the endometrium. *Menopause* 2001; **8**(5): 338-346.

15. Jacobs HS, Loeffler FE. Postmenopausal hormone replacement therapy. *BMJ* 1992; **305**(6866): 1403-8.

16. Lock M. Contested meanings of the menopause. *Lancet* 1991; **337**(8752): 1270-2.

17. Royal College of Obstetrics and Gynaecology. *Scientific Advisory Committee Opinion Paper 6: Alternatives to HRT for management of symptoms of the menopause.* London: RCOG, May 2006.

18. Rossouw JE, Anderson GL, Prentice RL. (Division of Women's Health Initiative). Risks and benefits of estrogen plus progestin in healthy postmenopausal women: principal results From the Women's Health Initiative randomized controlled trial. *JAMA* 2002; **288**(3): 321-33.

19. Stadberg E, Mattsson LA, Milsom I. Factors associated with climacteric symptoms and the use of hormone replacement therapy. *Acta Obstet Gynecol Scand* 2000; **79**(4): 286-292.

20. Wilbush J. Climacteric disorders: historical perspectives. In: Studd JWW, Whitehead MI (eds). *The Menopause*. Oxford: Blackwell Scientific Publications, 1988. pp 1-14.

21. Wilson RCD. *Understanding HRT and the menopause*. London: Consumers' Association and Hodder and Stoughton, 1992.

Natural Menopause

22. Chiechi LM, Putignano G, Guerra V, *et al*. The effect of a soya rich diet on the vaginal epithelium in post menopause: a randomized double blind trial. *Maturitas* 2003; **45**(4): 241-6.

23. Cline JM, Paschold JC, Anthony MS, Obasanjo IO, Adams MR. Effects of hormonal therapies and dietary soya phytoestrogens on vaginal cytology in surgically postmenopausal macaques. *Fertil Steril* 1996; **65**(5): 1031-5.

24. Craig WJ. Phytochemicals: guardians of our health. *J Am Diet Assoc* 1997: **97**(10 Suppl 2): 199-204.

25. Komesaroff PA, Black CV, Cable V, Sudhir K. Effects of wild yam extract on menopausal symptoms, lipids and sex hormones in healthy postmenopausal women. *Climacteric* 2001; **4**(2): 144-50.

26. Medicines and Healthcare Products Regulatory Agency, Committee on Safety of Medicines. Black cohosh (cimicifuga racemosa) and hepatotoxicity. In: *Current Problems in Pharmacovigilence, vol 30, page 10*. 2004. (www.formulary.cht.nhs.uk/pdf,_doc_files_etc/CSM/cp_2004_10.pdf).

27. Morelli V, Naquin C. Alternative therapies for traditional disease states: menopause. *Am Fam Physician* 2002; **66**(1): 129-134.

28. The role of isoflavones in menopausal health: consensus opinion of the North American Menopause Society. *Menopause* 2000: **7**(4): 215-229.

29. Treatment of menopause-associated vasomotor symptoms: position statement of the North American Menopause Society. *Menopause* 2004; **11**(1): 11-33.

30. Uesugi T, Toda T, Okuhira T, Chen JT. Evidence of estrogenic effect by the three-month-intervention of isoflavone on vaginal maturation and bone metabolism in early postmenopausal women. *Endocr J* 2003; **50**(5): 613-9.

31. Wilcox G, Wahlqvist ML, Burger HG, Medley G. Oestrogenic effects of plant foods in postmenopausal women. *BMJ* 1990; **301**(6757); 905-6.

Phytoestrogens

32. Adlercreutz H, Hamalainen E, Gorbach S, Goldin B. Dietary phyto-estrogens and the menopause in Japan. *Lancet* 1992; **339**(8803): 1233.

33. Adlercreutz H, Honjo H, Higashi A. Urinary excretion of lignans and isoflavonoid phytoestrogens in Japanese men and women consuming a traditional Japanese diet. *Am J Clin Nutr* 1991; **54**(6): 1093-1100.

34. Anderson JW, Johnstone BM, Cook-Newell ME. Meta-analysis of the effects of soya protein intake on serum lipids. *N Engl J Med* 1995; **333**(5): 276-82.

35. Appling S, Kelly K, Allen J. Impact of soya on menopausal symptoms. Orlando, Florida: Southern Nursing Research Society (SNRS) 17th Annual Conference, February 2003.

36. Badger TM, Ronis MJ, Hakkak R, Rowlands JC, Korourian S. The health consequences of early soya consumption. *J Nutr* 2002; **132**(3): 559S-565S.

37. Balk E, Chung M, Chew P, *et al*. Effects of soya on health outcomes. *Evid Rep Technol Assess (Summ)* 2005; **126**: 1-8.

38. Barnes S. Soya isoflavones - phytoestrogens and what else? *J Nutr* 2004; **134**(5): 1225S-1228S.

39. Brown BD, Thomas W, Hutchins A, Martini MC, Slavin JL. Types of dietary fat and soya minimally affect hormones and biomarkers associated with breast cancer risk in premenopausal women. *Nutr Cancer* 2002; **43**(1): 22-30.

40. Bryant M, Cassidy A, Hill C, *et al*. Effect of consumption of soya isoflavones on behavioural, somatic and affective symptoms in women with premenstrual syndrome. *Br J Nutr* 2005; **93**(5): 731-9.

41. Brzezinski A, Adlercreutz H, Shaoul R, *et al*. Short-term effects of phytoestrogen-rich diet on postmenopausal women. *J North Am Menopause Soc* 1997; **4**: 89-94.

42. Chacko BK, Chandler RT, Mundhekar A. Revealing anti-inflammatory mechanisms of soya isoflavones by flow: modulation of leukocyte-endothelial cell interactions. *Am J Physiol Heart Circ Physiol* 2005; **289**(2): H908-15.

43. Dwyer JT, Goldin BR, Saul N, *et al*. Tofu and soya drinks contain phytoestrogens. *J Am Diet Assoc* 1994: **94**(7): 739-743.

44. Faure ED, Chantre P, Mares P. Effects of a standardized soya extract on hot flushes: a multicentre, double-blind, randomized, placebo-controlled study. *Menopause* 2002; **9**(5): 329-34.

45. Hall WL, Vafeiadou K, Hallund J, *et al*. Soya-isoflavone-enriched foods and inflammatory biomarkers of cardiovascular disease risk in postmenopausal women: interactions with genotype and equol production. *Am J Clin Nutr* 2005; **82**(6): 1260-1268.

46. Han KK, Soares JM Jr, Haidar MA, de Lima GR, Baracat EC. Benefits of soya isoflavone therapeutic regimen on menopausal symptoms. *Obstet Gynecol* 2002; **99**(3): 389-94.

47. Joannou GE, Kelly GE, Reeder AY, Waring M, Nelson C. A urinary profile study of dietary phytoestrogens. The identification and mode of metabolism of new isoflavonoids. *J Steroid Biochem Mol Biol* 1995; **54**(3-4): 167-84.

48. Knight DC, Eden JA. Phtyestrogens - a short review. *Maturitas*. 1995; **22**(3): 165-75.

49. Kurzer MS, Xu X. Dietary phytoestrogens. *Annu Rev Nutr* 1997; **17**: 353-81.

50. Kurzer MS. Hormonal effects of soya in premenopausal women and men. *J Nutr* 2002; **132**(3): 570S-573S.

51. Kurzer MS, *et al* Soya isoflavones decrease hot-flash frequency: a meta-analysis of studies examining soya protein, soyafood, and soya isoflavones. Orlando, Florida: Fifth International Symposium on the Role of Soya in Preventing and Treating Chronic Disease, Sept 21-24 2003.

52. Lien LL, Lein EJ. Hormone therapy and phytoestrogens. *J Clin Pharm Ther* 1996; **21**(2): 101-11.

53. Markiewicz L, Garey J, Adlercreutz H, Gurpide E. In vitro bioassays of non-steroidal phytoestrogens. *J Steroid Biochem Molec Biol* 1993; **45**(5): 399-405.

54. Martin ME, Haourigui M, Pelissero C, Benassayag C, Nunez EA. Interactions between phytoestrogens and human sex steroid binding protein. *Life Sci* 1996; **58**(5): 429-36.

55. Mazur W. Phytoestrogen content in foods. *Baillièr's Clin Endocrinol Metab* 1998; **12**(4): 729-42.

56. Messina M. Soyafoods and soyabean phyto-oestrogens (isoflavones) as possible alternatives to hormone replacement therapy (HRT). *Eur J Cancer* 2000; **36**(4): S71-S72.

57. Messina M, Hughes C. Efficacy of soyafoods and soyabean isoflavone supplements for alleviating menopausal symptoms is positively related to initial hot flush frequency. *J Med Food* 2003; **6**(1): 1-11.

58. Messina M, Messina V. Provisional recommended soya protein and isoflavone intakes for healthy adults: rationale. *Nutr Today* 2003; **38**(3): 100-9.

59. Miksicek RJ. Commonly occurring plant flavonoids have estrogenic activity. Mol Pharmocol 1993; **44**(1): 37-43.

60. Nagata C, Shimizu H, Takami R, *et al*. Serum concentrations of estradiol and dehydroepiandrosterone sulfate and soya product intake in relation to psychologic well-being in peri- and postmenopausal Japanese women. *Metabolism* 2000; **49**(12): 1561-4.

61. Nagata C, Takatsuka N, Kawakami N, Shimizu H. Soya product intake and hot flashes in Japanese women: results from a community-based prospective study. *Am J Epidemiol* 2001; **153**(8): 790-793.

62. Petri NE, Nahas NJ, de Luca L, *et al*. Benefits of soya germ isoflavones in postmenopausal women with contraindication for conventional hormone replacement therapy. *Maturitas* 2004; **48**(4): 372-80.

63. Potter JD, Steinmetz K. Vegetables, fruit and phytoestrogens as preventive agents. *IARC Sci Publications* 1996; **139**: 61-90.

64. Reinli K, Block G. Phytoestrogen content of foods - a compendium of literature values. *Nutr Cancer* 1996; **26**(2): 123-148.

65. Ruiz-Larrea MB, Mohan AR, Paganga G, *et al*. Antioxidant activity of phytoestrogenic isoflavones. *Free Radic Res* 1997; **26**(1): 63-70.

66. Sacks F, Lichtenstein A, Van Horn L, *et al*. Soya protein, isoflavones and cardiovascular health: an American Heart Association Science Advisory for professionals from the Nutrition Committee. *Circulation* 2006; **113**(7): 1034-1044.

67. Scambia G, Mango D, Signorile PG, *et al*. Clinical effects of a standardised soya extract in postmenopausal women: a pilot study. *Menopause* 2000; **7**(2): 105-11.

68. Setchell KDR. Naturally occurring non-steroidal estrogens of dietary origin. In: McLachlan JA (ed). *Estrogens in the environment: influences on development*. New York: Elsevier, 1985: 69-83.

69. Setchell KD, Brown NM, Lydeking-Olsen E. The clinical importance of the metabolite equol - a clue to the effectiveness of soya and its isoflavones. *J Nutr* 2002; **132**(12): 3577-84.

70. Setchell KD. Phytoestrogens: the biochemistry, physiology and implications for human health of soya isoflavones. *Am J Clin Nutr* 1998; **68**(6 suppl): 1333S-1346S.

71. Somekawa Y, Chiguchi M, Ishibashi T, Aso T. Soya intake related to menopausal symptoms, serum lipids, and bone mineral density in postmenopausal Japanese women. *Obstet Gynecol* 2001; **97**(1): 109-115.

72. St Clair RW. Estrogens and atherosclerosis: phytoestrogens and selective estrogen receptor modulators. *Curr Opin Lipidol* 1998; **9**(5): 457-63.

73. Tham DM, Gardner CD, Haskell WL. Potential health benefits of dietary phytoestrogens: a review of the clinical, epidemiological and mechanistic evidence. *J Clin Endocrinol Metab* 1998; **83**(7): 2223-2235.

74. Wang HJ, Murphy PA. Isoflavone content in commercial soyabean foods. *J Agr Food Chem* 1994; **42**: 1666-73

Lignans

75. Borriello SP, Setchell KD, Axelson M, Lawson AM. Production and metabolism of lignans by the human faecal flora. *J Appl Bacteriol* 1985; **58**(1): 37-43.

76. Franco OH, Burger H, Lebrun CE, *et al*. Higher dietary intake of lignans is associated with better cognitive performance in postmenopausal women. *J Nutr* 2005; **135**(5): 1190-1195.

77. Lemay A, Dodin S, Kadri N, Jacques H, Forest JC. Flaxseed dietary supplement versus hormone replacement therapy in hypercholesterolemic menopausal women. *Obstet Gynecol* 2002; **100**(3): 495-504.

78. Obormeyer WR, Warner C, Casey RE, Musser S. Flaxseed lignans isolation, metabolism and biological effects. *FASEB J* 1993; **7**(Abstract 4965).

79. Setchell KD, Lawson AM, Mitchell FL, *et al*. Lignans in man and in animal species. *Nature* 1980; **287**(5784); 740-742.

80. Thompson LU, Robb P, Serraino M, Cheung F. Mammalian lignan production from various foods. *Nutr Cancer* 1991; **16**(1): 43-52.

General Diet

81. Adlercreutz H, Fotsis T, Bannwart C, *et al*. Assay of lignans and phytoestrogens in urine of women and in cow's milk by GC/MS (SIM) In: Todd JFJ (ed). Advances in Mass Spectrometry-*85*. Tenth International Mass Spectrometry Conference Chichester: John Wiley, 1985; 661-2.

82. Campagnoli C, Abba C, Ambroggio S, *et al*. Polyunsaturated fatty acids (PUFAs) might reduce hot flushes: an indication from two controlled trials on soya isoflavones alone and with a PUFA supplement. *Maturitas* 2005; **51**(2): 127-34.

83. Hutchins AM, Lampe JW, Martini MS, Campbell DR, Slavin JL. Vegetables, fruits and legumes: effect on urinary isoflavanoid phytoestrogen and lignan excretion. *J Am Diet Assoc* 1995: **95**(7): 769-74.

84. Albert A, Altabre G, Baro F, *et al*. Efficacy and safety of a phytoestrogen preparation derived from Glycine max (L.) Merr in climacteric symptomatology: a multicentric, open, prospective and non-randomized trial. *Phytomedicine* 2002; **9**(2): 85-92.

85. Albertazzi P, Pansini F, Bonaccorsi G, *et al*. The effect of dietary soya supplementation on hot flushes. *Obstet Gynecol* 1998; **91**(1): 6-11.

86. Atkinson C, Warren RM, Sala E, *et al*. Red-clover-derived isoflavones and mammographic breast density: a double-blind, randomized, placebo-controlled trial. *Breast Cancer Res* 2004; **6**(3): R170-9.

87. Erkkola R, Yang B. Sea buckthorn oils: towards healthy mucous membranes. *AgroFood industry hi-tech* 2003; **3**: 53-57.

88. Faure ED, Chantre P, Mares P. Effects of a standardized soya extract on hot flushes: a multicentre double-blind, randomized, placebo-controlled study. *Menopause* 2002; **9**(5): 329-334.

89. Husband AJ. Phytoestrogens and menopause. Published evidence supports a role for phytoestrogens in menopause. *BMJ* 2002; **324**(7328): 52.

90. Husband AJ. Red Clover isoflavone supplements: safety and pharmacokinetics. *J Br Menopause Soc* 2001; **Suppl1**: 4-7.

91. Jeri AR. The use of an isoflavone supplement to relieve hot flushes. *The Female Patient* 2002; **27**: 35-37.

92. Nachtigall LB, Nachtigall MJ, Nachtigall LE. Non-prescription alternatives to hormone replacement therapy. *The Female Patient* 1999; **24**: 59.

93. Punnonen R, Lukola A. Oestrogen-like effect of ginseng. *BMJ* 1980; **281**(6248): 1110.

94. Thompson Coon J, Pittler MH, Ernst E. The role of red clover (Trifolium pratense) isoflavones in women's reproductive health: a systematic review and meta-analysis of randomised clinical trials. *Focus Altern Complement Ther* 2003; **8**: 544.

95. Van de Weijer PH, Barentsen R. Isoflavones from red clover (Promensil) significantly reduce menopausal hot flush symptoms compared with placebo. *Maturitas* 2002; **42**(3): 187-93.

96. Woods R, Whitehead M. Effects of red clover isoflavones (promensil) versus placebo on uterine endometrium, vaginal maturation index and the uterine artery in healthy postmenopausal women. *J Br Menopause Soc* 2003; **SupplS2**: 33.

97. Yang B, Kallio H. Composition and physiological effects of sea buckthorn lipids. *Trends in Food Sci Technol* 2002; **13**: 160-167.

98. Yang B, Kallio H. Physiological effects of sea buckthorn (Hippophaë rhamnoides) fruit pulp and seed oils. In: Singh V, Yang B, Kallio H, *et al* (eds). *Seabuckthorn (Hippophaë L). A Multipurpose Wonder Plant. Vol II: Biochemistry and Pharmacology.* New Delhi, India: Dya Publishing House, pp 363-389.

99. Yang B. *Lipophilic components of sea buckthorn (Hippophaë rhamnoides) seeds and berries and physiological effects of sea buckthorn oils.* Finland: University of Turku, 2001.

100. Yang B, Kallio HP. Fatty acid composition of lipids in sea buckthorn (Hippophaë rhamnoides L.) berries of different origins. *J Agric Food Chem* 2001; **49**(4): 1939-1947.

Exercise and Relaxation

101. Cowan MM, Gregory LW. Responses of pre- and postmenopausal females to aerobic conditioning. *Med Sci Sports Exerc* 1985; **17**(1): 138-43.

102. Greist JH, Klein MH, Eischens RR, *et al.* Running as treatment for depression. *Compr Psychiatry*, 1979; **20**(1): 41-54.

103. Greendale GA, Gold GB. Lifestyle factors: are they related to vasomotor symptoms and do they modify the effectiveness or side effects of hormone therapy? *Am J Med* 2005; **118**(Suppl 12B): 148-54.

104. Ivarsson T, Spetz AL, Hammar M. Physical exercise and vasomotor symptoms in postmenopausal women. *Maturitas* 1998; **29**(2): 139-146.

105. Lindh-Astrand L, Nedstrand E, Wyon Y, Hammar M. Vasomotor symptoms and quality of life in previously sedentary postmenopausal women randomised to physical activity or estrogen therapy. *Maturitas* 2004; **48**(2): 97-105.

106. Martin D, Notelovitz M. Effects of aerobic training on bone mineral density of postmenopausal women. *J. Bone Miner Res* 1993; **8**(8): 931-6.

107. Nedstrand E, Wijma K, Wyon Y, Hammar M. Applied relaxation and oral estradiol treatment of vasomotor symptoms in postmenopausal women. *Maturitas* 2005; **51**(2): 154-62.

Complementary Therapies

108. Thompson EA, Reilly D. The homeopathic approach to the treatment of symptoms of oestrogen withdrawal in breast cancer patients. A prospective observational study. *Homeopathy* 2003; **92**(3): 131-4.

109. Wyon Y, Wijma K, Nedstrand E, Hammar M. A comparison of acupuncture and oral estradiol treatment of vasomotor symptoms in postmenopausal women. *Climacteric* 2004; **7**(2): 153-64.

Heart Disease

110. Baum JA, Teng H, Erdman JW Jr, *et al*. Long-term intake of soya protein improves blood lipid profiles and increases mononuclear cell low-density-lipoprotein receptor messenger RNA in hypercholesterolemic, postmenopausal women. *Am J Clin Nutr* 1998; **68**(3): 545-551.

111. Cassidy A, Griffin B. Phyto-estrogens: a potential role in the prevention of CHD? *Proc Nutr Soc* 1999; **58**(1): 193-199.

112. Chen CY, Bakhiet RM, Hart V, Holtzmann G. Isoflavones improve plasma homocysteine status and antioxidant defense system in healthy young men at rest but do not ameliorate oxidative stress induced by 80% VO2pk exercise. *Ann Nutr Metab* 2005; **49**(1): 33-41.

113. Dewailly E, Blanchet C, Gingras S, Lemieux S, Holub BJ. Cardiovascular disease risk factors and n-3 fatty acid status in the adult population of James Bay Cree. *Am J Clin Nutr* 2002; **76**(1): 85-92.

114. Erdman JW Jr. AHA Science Advisory: Soya protein and cardiovascular disease: a statement for healthcare professionals from the Nutrition Committee of the AHA. *Circulation* 2000; **102**(20): 2555-9.

115. Erkkila AT, Lehto S, Pyorala K, Uusitupa MI. n-3 Fatty acids and 5-y risks of death and cardiovascular disease events in patients with coronary artery disease. *Am J Clin Nutr* 2003; **78**(1): 65-71.

116. Food Labeling: Health Claims; Soya Protein and Coronary Heart Disease. In: *Federal Register* 1999: **64**(206): 57699-733.

117. Food and Drug Administration, US Department of Health and Human Services. *FDA approves new health claim for soya protein and coronary heart disease: FDA talk paper*. USA: FDA, October 20, 1999: T99-48.

118. Geleijnse JM, Giltay EJ, Grobbee DE, Donders AR, Kok FJ. Blood pressure response to fish oil supplementation: metaregression analysis of randomized trials. *J Hypertens* 2002; **20**(8): 1493-9.

119. Greendale GA, Gold EB. Lifestyle factors: are they related to vasomotor symptoms and do they modify the effectiveness or side effects of hormone therapy? *Am J Med* 2005; **118**(Suppl 12B):148-54.

120. Haq IU, Jackson PR, Yeo WW, Ramsay LE. Sheffield risk and treatment table for cholesterol lowering for primary prevention of coronary heart disease. *Lancet* 1995; **346**(8988): 1467-1471.

121. Howes JB, Tran D, Brillante D, Howes LG. Effects of dietary supplementation with isoflavones from red clover on ambulatory blood pressure and endothelial function in postmenopausal type 2 diabetes. *Diabetes Obes Metab* 2003; **5**(5): 325-32.

122. Jenkins DJ, Kendall CW, Jackson CJ, *et al.* Effects of high- and low-isoflavone soyafoods on blood lipids, oxidized LDL, homocysteine, and blood pressure in hyperlipidemic men and women. *Am J Clin Nutr* 2002; **76**(2): 365-72.

123. Jeri A. Effects of isoflavone phytoestrogens on lipid profile in postmenopausal Peruvian Women. Presented at the 10th World Congress on the Menopause, Berlin, June 2002.

124. Marchioli R, Schweiger C, Tavazzi L, Valagussa F. Efficacy of n-3 polyunsaturated fatty acids after myocardial infarction: results of GISSI-Prevenzione trial. Gruppo Italiano per lo Studio della Sopravvivenza nell'Infarto Miocardico. *Lipids* 2001; **36**(Suppl): S119-26.

125. Mitsuyoshi K, Hiramatsu Y, Takata T, *et al.* Effects of eicosapentaenoic acid on lipid metabolism in obesity treatment. *Obes Surg* 1991; **1**(2): 165-169.

126. Nestel P. Fish oil fatty acids beneficially modulate vascular function. *World Rev Nutr Diet* 2001; **88**: 86-9.

127. Nestel P, Pomeroy S, Kay S, *et al.* Isoflavones from red clover improve systemic arterial compliance but not plasma lipids in menopausal women. *J Clin Endocrinol Metab* 1999; **84**(3): 895-8.

128. Nestel P, Shige H, Pomeroy S, *et al.* The n-3 fatty acids eicosapentaenoic acid and docosahexaenoic acid increase systemic arterial compliance in humans. *Am J Clin Nutr* 2002; **76**(2): 326-30.

129. Okuda N, Ueshima H, Okayama A, *et al.* Relation of long chain n-3 polyunsaturated fatty acid intake to serum high density lipoprotein cholesterol among Japanese men in Japan and Japanese-American men in Hawaii: the interlipid study. *Atherosclerosis* 2005; **178**(2): 371-9.

130. Okumura T, Fujioka Y, Morimoto S, *et al*. Eicosapentaenoic acid improves endothelial function in hypertriglyceridemic subjects despite increased lipid oxidizability. *Am J Med Sci* 2002; **324**(5): 247-53.

131. Steinberg FM, Guthrie NL, Villablanca AC, Kumar K, Murray MJ. Soya protein with isoflavones has favorable effects on endothelial function that are independent of lipid and antioxidant effects in healthy postmenopausal women. *Am J Clin Nutr* 2003; **78**(1): 123-30.

132. Tagawa T, Hirooka Y, Shimokawa H, *et al*. Long-term treatment with eicosapentaenoic acid improves exercise-induced vasodilation in patients with coronary artery disease. *Hypertens Res* 2002; **25**(6): 823-9.

133. Teede HJ, McGrath BP, deSilva L, *et al*. Isoflavones reduce arterial stiffness: a placebo-controlled study in men and postmenopausal women. *Arterioscler Thromb Vasc Biol* 2003; **23**(6): 1066-71.

134. Thies F, Garry JM, Yaqoob P, *et al*. Association of n-3 polyunsaturated fatty acids with stability of 4therosclerotic plaques: a randomised controlled trial. *Lancet* 2003; **361**(9356): 477-85.

135. Von Schacky C. The role of omega-3 fatty acids in cardiovascular disease. *Curr Atheroscler Rep* 2003; **5**(2): 139-45.

136. Washburn S, Burke GL, Morgan T, Anthony M. Effect of soya protein supplementation on serum lipoproteins, blood pressure and menopausal symptoms in perimenopausal women. *Menopause* 1999; **6**(1): 7-13.

137. Yu Z, Zhang G, Zhao H. Effects of puerariae isoflavone on blood viscosity, thrombosis and platelet function. *Zhong Yao Cai* 1997; **20**(9): 468-9.

138. Zhan S, Ho SC. Meta-analysis of the effects of soya protein containing isoflavones on the lipid profile. *Am J Clin Nutr* 2005; **81**(2): 397-408.

Cholesterol

139. Johnston IM, James R. *Flaxseed (linseed) oil and the power of omega-3*. McGraw Hill. 1995.

Osteoporosis / Post Menopause

140. Arjmandi BH, Khalil DA, Smith BJ, *et al*. Soya protein has a greater effect on bone in postmenopausal women not on hormone replacement therapy, as evidenced by reducing bone resorption and urinary calcium excretion. *J Clin Endocrinol Metab* 2003; **88**(3): 1048-54.

141. Atkinson C, Compston JE, Day NE, Dowsett M, Bingham SA. The effects of phytoestrogen isoflavones on bone density in women: a double-blind, randomized, placebo-controlled trial. *Am J Clin Nutr* 2004; **79**(2): 326-33.

142. Blumsohn A, Herrington K, Hannon RA, *et al*. The effect of calcium supplementation on the circadian rhythm of bone resorption. *J Clin Endocrinol Metab* 1994; **79**(3): 730-35.

143. Bonaiuti D, Shea B, Lovine R, *et al*. Exercise for preventing and treating osteoporosis in postmenopausal women (review). The Cochrane Library: 4. Chichester: John Wiley, 2004.

144. Chen YM, Ho SC, Lam SS, Ho SS, Woo JL. Beneficial effect of soya isoflavones on bone mineral content was modified by years since menopause, body weight, and calcium intake: a double-blind, randomized, controlled trial. *Menopause* 2004; **11**(3): 246-54.

145. Berg G, Hammar M (eds). *The modern management of the menopause*. New York; London: Parthenon Publishing, 1994.

146. Dixon AS. Non-hormonal treatment of osteoporosis. *BMJ* 1983; **286**(6370): 999-1000.

147. Ettinger B, Grady D. The waning effect of postmenopausal estrogen therapy on osteoporosis. *N Engl J Med*, 1993; **329**(16): 1141-6.

148. Horiuchi T, Onouchi T, Takahashi M, Ito H, Orino H. Effect of soya protein on bone metabolism in postmenopausal Japanese women. *Osteoporos Int* 2000; **11**(8): 721-4.

149. Kanis JA, Johnell O, Gullberg B, *et al*. Evidence for efficacy of drugs affecting bone metabolism in preventing hip fracture. *BMJ* 1992; **305**(6862): 1124-8.

150. Mei J, Yeung SS, Kung AW. High dietary phytoestrogen intake is associated with higher bone mineral density in postmenopausal but not premenopausal women. *J Clin Endocrinol Metab* 2001; **86**(11): 5217-21.

151. Messina M, Messina V. Soyafoods, soyabean isoflavones and bone health: a brief overview. *J Ren Nutr* 2000; **10**(2): 63-8.

152. Morabito N, Crisafulli A, Vergara C, *et al*. Effects of genistein and hormone-replacement therapy on bone loss in early postmenopausal women: a randomized double-blind placebo-controlled study. *J Bone Miner Res* 2002; **17**(10): 1904-12.

153. Peel N, Eastell R. Osteoporosis. *BMJ* 1995; **310**(6985); 989-92.

154. Scheiber MD, Liu JH, Subbiah MT, Rebar RW, Setchell KD. Dietary inclusion of whole soya foods results in significant reductions in clinical risk factors for osteoporosis and cardiovascular disease in normal postmenopausal women. *Menopause* 2001; **8**(5): 384-92.

155. Setchell KD, Lydeking-Olsen E. Dietary phytoestrogens and their effect on bone: evidence from in vitro and in vivo, human observational, and dietary intervention studies. *Am J Clin Nutr* 2003; **78**(3 Suppl): 593S-609S.

156. Studd JWW, Whitehead MI (eds). *The Menopause*. Oxford: Blackwell Scientific Publications, 1988.

157. Tsunenari T, Yamada S, Kawakatsu M, Negishi H, Tsutsumi M. Menopause-related changes in bone mineral density in Japaene women: a longitudinal study on lumbar spine and proximal femur. *Calcif Tissue Int* 1995; **56**(1): 5-10.

158. Van Papendorp DH, Coetzer H, Kruger MC. Biochemical profile of osteoporotic patients on essential fatty acid supplementation. *Nutr Res* 1995; **15**: 325-34.

159. Wilcox G, Wahlqvist ML, Burger HG, Medley G. Oestrogenic effects of plant foods in postmenopausal women. *BMJ* 1990; **301**(6757): 905.

160. WHO Study Group. *Assessment of fracture risk and its application to screening for postmenopausal osteoporosis*. World Health Organization, 1994; 843: 11-3.

Memory

161. Duffy R, Wiseman H, File SE. Improved cognitive function in postmenopausal women after 12 weeks of consumption of a soya extract containing isoflavones. *Pharmacol Biochem Behav* 2003; **75**(3): 721-9.

162. Elsabagh S, Hartley DE, File SE. Limited cognitive benefits in Stage +2 postmenopausal women after six weeks of treatment with Ginkgo biloba. *J Psychopharmacol* 2005; **19**(2): 173-9.

163. File SE, Jarrett N, Fluck E, *et al*. Eating soya improves human memory. *Psychopharmacology* 2001; **157**(4): 430-436.

164. Kritz-Silverstein D, Von Muhlen D, Barrett-Connor E, Bressel MA. Isoflavones and cognitive function in older women: the soya and postmenopausal health in aging (SOPHIA) study. *Menopause* 2003; **10**(3): 196-202.

165. Atkinson C, Warren RM, Sala E, *et al*. Red-clover-derived isoflavones and mammographic breast density: a double-blind, randomized, placebo-controlled trial [ISRCTN42940165]. *Breast Cancer Res* 2004; **6**(3): R170-9.

166. Boyd NF, Lockwood GA, Martin LJ, *et al*. Mammographic density as a marker of susceptibility to breast cancer: a hypothesis. *IARC Sci Publ* 2001; **154**: 163-9.

167. Fleming RM. What effect, if any, does soya protein have on breast tissue? *Integr Cancer Ther* 2003; **2**(3): 225-8.

168. Goodman MT, Wilkens LR, Hankin JH, *et al*. Association of soya and fiber consumption with the risk of endometrial cancer. *Am J Epidemiol* 1997; **146**(4): 294-306.

169. Horn-Ross PL, John EM, Canchola AJ, Stewart SL, Lee MM. Phytoestrogen intake and endometrial cancer risk. *J Natl Cancer Inst* 2003; **95**(15): 1158-64.

170. Ingram DM Hickling C, West L, Mahe LJ, Dunbar PM. A double-blind randomized controlled trial of isoflavones in the treatment of cyclical mastalgia. *Breast* 2002; **11**(2): 170-174.

171. Lu LJ, Anderson KE, Grady JJ, Kohen F, Nagamani M. Decreased ovarian hormones during a soya diet: implications for breast cancer prevention. *Cancer Res* 2000; **60**(15): 4112-21.

172. Maskarinec G, Murphy S, Franke AA, *et al*. The effects of a nutritional intervention with soyafoods on markers of breast cancer risk. *Exp Biol 2004*; **Abstract 728**: 4.

173. Maskarinec G, Williams AE, Carlin L. Mammographic densities in a one-year isoflavone intervention. *Eur J Cancer Prev* 2003; **12**(2):165-9.

174. Wu AH, Stanczyk FZ, Seow A, Lee HP, Yu MC. Soya intake and other lifestyle determinants of serum estrogen levels among postmenopausal Chinese women in Singapore. *Cancer Epidemiol Biomarkers Prev* 2002; **11**(9): 844-51.

175. Xu X, Duncan AM, Wangen KE, Kurzer MS. Soya consumption alters endogenous estrogen metabolism in postmenopausal women. *Cancer Epidemiol Biomarkers Prev* 2000; **9**(8): 781-6.

176. Beiler JS, Zhu K, Hunter S, *et al*. A case-control study of menstrual factors in relation to breast cancer risk in African-American women. *J Natl Med Assoc* 2003; **95**(10): 930-8.

177. den Tonkelaar I, de Waard F. Regularity and length of menstrual cycles in women aged 41-46 in relation to breast cancer risk: results from the DOM-project. *Breast Cancer Res Treat* 1996; **38**(3): 253-8.

178. Huang Y, Cao S, Nagamani M, *et al*. 2005. Decreased circulating levels of tumor necrosis factor-alpha in postmenopausal women during consumption of soya-containing isoflavones. *J Clin Endocrinol Metab* 2005; **90**(7): 3956-62.

179. Jakes RW, Duffy SW, Ng FC, *et al*. Mammographic parenchymal patterns and self-reported soya intake in Singapore Chinese women. *Cancer Epidemiol Biomarkers Prev* 2002; **11**(7): 608-613.

180. Kumar NB, Cantor A, Allen K, Riccardi D, Cox CE. The specific role of isoflavones on estrogen metabolism in premenopausal women. *Cancer* 2002; **94**(4): 1166-74.

181. Magee PJ, McGlynn H, Rowland IR. Differential effects of isoflavones and lignans on invasiveness of MDA-MB-231 breast cancer cells in vitro. *Cancer Lett* 2004; **208**(1): 35-41.

182. Parkin DM (ed). Cancer incidence in five continents. Lyon: International Agency for Research on Cancer, 1997.

183. Peterson TG, Ji GP, Kirk M, *et al*. Metabolism of the isoflavones genistein and biochanin A in human breast cancer cell lines. *Am J Clin Nutr* 1998; **68**(6 Suppl): 1505S-1511S.

184. Pfeiffer E, Treiling CR, Hoehle SI, Metzler M. Isoflavones modulate the glucuronidation of estradiol in human liver microsomes. *Carcinogenesis* 2005; **26**(12): 2172-8.

185. Takezaki T, Hirose K, Inoue M, et al. Risk factors of thyroid cancer among women in Tokai, Japan. *J Epidemiol* 1996; **6**(3): 140-7.

186. Valachovicova T, Slivova V, Bergman H, Shuherk J, Sliva D. Soya isoflavones suppress invasiveness of breast cancer cells by the inhibition of NF-kappaB/AP-1-dependent and -independent pathways. *Int J Oncol* 2004; **25**(5): 1389-95.

187. Yamamoto S, Sobue T, Kobayashi M, Sasaki S, Tsugane S. Soya, isoflavones, and breast cancer risk in Japan. *J Natl Cancer Inst* 2003; **95**(12): 906-13.

188. Yin F, Giuliano AE, Van Herle AJ. Growth inhibitory effects of flavonoids in human thyroid cancer cell lines. *Thyroid* 1999; **9**(4): 369-76.

189. Xu X, Duncan AM, Merz BE, Kurzer MS. Effects of soya isoflavones on estrogen and phytoestrogen metabolism in premenopausal women. *Cancer Epidemiol Biomarkers Prev* 1998; **7**(12): 1101-08.

Thyroid Function

190. Bruce B, Messina M, Spiller GA. Isoflavone supplements do not affect thyroid function in iodine-replete postmenopausal women. *J Med Food* 2003; **6**(4): 309-16.

191. Doerge DR, Sheehan DM. Goitrogenic and estrogenic activity of soya isoflavones. *Environ Health Perspect* 2002; **110**(Suppl 3): 349-53.

192. Duncan AM, Merz PE, Xu X, *et al*. Soya isoflavones exert modest hormonal effects in premenopausal women. *J Clin Endocrinol Metab* 1999; **84**(1): 192-7.

193. Duncan AM, Underhill KE, Xu X, *et al*. Modest hormonal effects of soya isoflavones in postmenopausal women. *J Clin Endocrinol Metab* 1999; **84**(10): 3479-84.

194. Liel Y, Harman-Boehm I, Shany S. Evidence for a clinically important adverse effect of fiber-enriched diet on the bioavailability of levothyroxine in adult hypothyroid patients. *J Clin Endocrinol Metab* 1996; **81**(2): 857-9.

Menstrual Problems

195. Bryant M, Dye L, Hill C, Powell J, Talbot D, Cassidy A. Role of phytoestrogens for menstrual cycle symptoms. *J Nutr* 2003; **134**: 1282 (abstract).

196. Ferrante F, Fusco E, Calabresi P, Cupini LM. Phyto-oestrogens in the prophylaxis of menstrual migraine. *Clin Neuropharmacol* 2004; **27**(3): 137-40.

Ask Maryon Stewart
and
Natural Health Advisory Service
PO Box 117
Rottingdean
Brighton BN51 9BG
UNITED KINGDOM
Ph +44 (0) 1273 609699
Email enquiries@askmaryonstewart.com

Recommended Reading
Cruising Through the Menopause, Maryon Stewart, Vermilion
The Phyto Factor, Maryon Stewart, Vermilion
The Natural Health Bible, Maryon Stewart and Dr Alan Stewart, New Holland

Useful websites
www.askmaryonstewart.com
www.naturalmenopause.com
www.naturalhealthas.com

The NHAS have clinics and run a Telephone Consultation Service that has been helping menopausal women all over the world for the last 20 years.

Recommended books and supplements can be obtained from the online shop at
www.askmaryonstewart.com/member

mail order details

USA
Ask Maryon Stewart Ltd
c/o Aruis Marketing
780 E. Riverpark Ln
Boise ID 83706

Phone (800) 587-4513 (toll free)

Australia and New Zealand
Ask Maryon Stewart Ltd
PO Box 3300
Malaga 6945
Western Australia

Phone 1800 611744 (toll free)

United Kingdom
Ask Maryon Stewart Ltd
7 Park Crescent
London W1B 1PF

Phone 020 7107 0698

Canada
Ask Maryon Stewart Ltd
42 Maple Avenue
Barrie, Ontario
L4N 1R8

Phone   1800 526 9772 (toll free)